Aging Invisibly

Personal/Public Scholarship

VOLUME 13

The titles published in this series are listed at *brill.com/pepu*

Aging Invisibly

Championing Diversity in Scholarship on Growing Older with Chronic Illness

Edited by

Alexandra "Xan" C.H. Nowakowski and J.E. Sumerau

BRILL

LEIDEN | BOSTON

Cover illustration: iStock.com/Jorge Aguado Martin

All chapters in this book have undergone peer review.

Library of Congress Cataloging-in-Publication Data

Names: Nowakowski, Alexandra "Xan" C. H. editor. | Sumerau, J. E., editor.
Title: Aging invisibly : championing diversity in scholarship on growing older with chronic illness / edited by Alexandra "Xan" C.H. Nowakowski and J.E. Sumerau.
Description: Leiden ; Boston : Brill, [2024] | Series: Personal/public scholarship, 2542-9671 ; volume 13 | Includes bibliographical references.
Identifiers: LCCN 2024029903 (print) | LCCN 2024029904 (ebook) | ISBN 9789004708129 (hardback ; acid-free paper) | ISBN 9789004708112 (paperback ; acid-free paper) | ISBN 9789004708136 (e-book)
Subjects: LCSH: Chronic diseases. | Aging. | Chronically ill--Health and hygiene. | Older people--Health and hygiene.
Classification: LCC RA644.5 .A44 2024 (print) | LCC RA644.5 (ebook) | DDC 616/.044--dc23/eng/20240730
LC record available at https://lccn.loc.gov/2024029903
LC ebook record available at https://lccn.loc.gov/2024029904

Typeface for the Latin, Greek, and Cyrillic scripts: "Brill". See and download: brill.com/brill-typeface.

ISSN 2542-9671
ISBN 978-90-04-70811-2 (paperback)
ISBN 978-90-04-70812-9 (hardback)
ISBN 978-90-04-70813-6 (e-book)
DOI 10.1163/9789004708136

This book is printed on acid-free paper and produced in a sustainable manner.

For all those getting through this life unsung. We see you—and you matter.

Contents

Acknowledgements

Thank you to everyone at Brill for their support and consideration throughout the process of this book. No book, edited volume or otherwise, is completed without the insights and help of a collective people—we are grateful for the folks at Brill for all their support along the way. We especially appreciate John Bennett for bearing with us during the lengthy development process for this volume and all the challenges it brought. Here's to the fruits of our labors at last, truly ones of love at every turn.

Alexandra "Xan" Nowakowski would also like to thank J Sumerau for being another half in this project and all things. Here's to 13 years and many more of writing a great story together.

They are grateful to family of origin and choice who have nurtured their scholarship and impact at every turn, beginning with their parents Nancy Hayes and Richard Nowakowski—the original "paradox" who have inspired so much. Also to the one without a face who gave a life. Thank you to Nik Lampe for your massive heart and earnest team spirit. To Lain Mathers and Shay Phillips for enduring fellowship. And to PNV, an artist of influence who brings light into every shadow.

To Mercedes Kim, Sydney Allen, Kenneth Quinnell, Hillary Gross, Clare Gould, and Sarah Kelly for allyship in similar struggles and critical times. To Dominic Quagliozzi, Jes Davis, Kelsey Smith, April Biggs, Grant Manczuk, and Ela Castillo who share many of the very same ones.

They are grateful for colleagues in missions great and small. To Rob Glueckauf, Tomeka Norton-Brown, and Wanda Rodríguez-Donham who are true siblings in spirit. To Tiffaney Holcomb, Nicolette Castagna, LaVon Edgerton, Skyler Bastow, and Kate Kazmierski who keep the joy in the work. To Patricia Leavy and Shalen Lowell for constant uplifting of storytellers. To Ron Chenail, Adam Rosenthal, and Courtney Morales for keeping narrative firmly in research. To Kokos Markides, Bill Cockerham, and Jen Taylor-Cousar for unflagging support. To Kathy Charmaz and the torch she passed along.

To Carolyn Blue, Ramiz Kseri, Mike Nair-Collins, Joe Gabriel, Niharika Suchak, Cesar Rodriguez, Mary Gerend, Butch Mazumder, Greg Todd, Jessica De Leon, Stephen Chelko, Tyra Dark, Casey Rust, Gina Sutin, Antonio Terracciano, Shenifa Taite, Tana Welch, Scott Pickett, Cheryl Porter, Becky Carter, Lisa Gardner, and Nissa Askins for enduring solidarity in the good fight. To Bob Watson for being there when it mattered most. To Katie Graves, Brittny James, Sammy Goldfarb, Lacey Ritter, Chait Renduchintala, Davalda Bellot, Catherine García, Milica Jovanov, Josh Paredes, Kerly Lapaine, and Priscilla Morelli for collaborations of enlightenment old and new. To Regina Scott, Tai Smith, Sarah English, Amy Larsen, and Heather Gordon for making the rubber meet the road. To Mary Dailey and Charlie Ouimet, remembered and cherished.

Xan is also grateful to those who have mentored and supported them in leadership over the years. To Jill Quadagno, Miles Taylor, Terrence Hill, John Taylor, Neil Charness, Anne Barrett, Kathi Tillman, Irene Padavic, Ike Eberstein, and John Reynolds; to Bernadette West, Lois Grau, Derek Shendell, and Vicki Freedman; to Paul Katz, Lisa Granville, Heather Flynn, Ken Brummel-Smith, and Suzanne Johnson; to Mike Devine, Scott Helzer, Tommy Bowermeister, and Mike Smith; to Jay Fogarty, Alma Littles, Mike Muszynski, Joan Meek, and Mark Chaet; to Henry Carretta, Gail Bellamy, Jo Brown Speights, Jon Appelbaum, and George Rust; and to Dan Van Durme and Myra Hurt whose light shines on brightly.

To colleagues from FSU, UCF, Rutgers, USACFA, and more—not named but treasured just the same. To collaborators at CDC, HRSA, Columbia, and myriad nonprofits all the way back to SONJ. To friends all around the world, near and far, sick and well. To so many more for a thousand small gifts. The words don't feel like enough.

J. Sumerau would like to thank Xan Nowakowski for inviting them to join this project, and for their ongoing support on this and so many other research and literary projects over the past decade-plus of working and existing together in varied ways.

They also owe deep gratitude to the love, support, and challenges of long-time co-livers-and-writers-and-researchers including especially Nik Lampe, Lain Mathers, Shay Phillips, Pina Holway, Mandi Barringer, Eve Haydt, Dave Mercer, Kayte Branch, and Brandy Ferguson.

J also wishes to especially thank Irene Padavic, Douglas Schrock, Koji Ueno, Kim Davies, Patricia Leavy, Allen Scarboro, Katie Acosta, John Reynolds, Patricia Yancey Martin, and Dawne Moon for too many contributions to count as mentors and heroes informally and formally throughout their career.

Finally, we both wish to thank the contributors in this volume for a long and fulfilling process of creation, discovery, revisions, administration, and just plain old work toward the creation of this volume over the past few years and through the extra considerations created by pandemic experiences.

Illustrations

Figures

Table

Notes on Contributors

Nicholas B. DiCarlo

has an MSW from Hunter College, where they now teach decolonial approaches to social work practice in addition to their psychotherapy practice. They are a co-director of the Emancipatory Sciences Lab at UCSF and associate editor of Routledge's Aging & Society Series with Carroll Estes. Their next book *Dreaming Generations: Psychoanalytic Perspectives toward Emancipatory Gerontology* (forthcoming, Routledge) explores racialized fractures in the generational transmission of wisdom part and parcel to coloniality's oppressive, extractive strategy against the psyche's capacity for collectivity and resistance.

Angela Hunt

is a Health Educator with Hope and Help serving people recovering from substance abuse and addiction in the greater Orlando area. She serves on a number of community nonprofit boards, and provides information and support about many different health issues impacting people with a history of street drug use. These include Hepatitis C, HIV, other bloodborne infections, mental health, social support, harm reduction, medication assisted therapy, and more. She is also a proud advocate for transgender Floridians and champions gender justice in all of her work.

Ian M. Johnson

is currently an Assistant Professor at the University of Texas–San Antonio's College of Health, Community & Policy. Ian's research seeks housing and health justice for older adults. They are the primary investigator of the Research, Action & Supportive Care at Later-life for Unhoused Peoples (RASCAL-UP) Study, a partnership with UW Medicine Harborview's Mobile Homeless Palliative Care Outreach Team. Ian has a doctorate in Social Welfare and is a licensed social worker. He continues direct practice with older people and their networks of care, and teaches direct social work practice to emerging social workers.

Nat Jones

is now a resident of Obstetrics and Gynecology at UPMC in Pittsburgh, PA. There, they actively provide gender-affirming care with the overarching goal of helping to create a dedicated gender care clinic within the OBGYN department. Their research foci include LGBTQ+ cancer health disparities, intersex patient advocacy, and gender diverse mental health needs. In their spare time, Dr. Jones likes to take care of house plants, exercise with friends, and read science fiction.

Kristen D. Krause
is an instructor of urban health in the Department of Urban-Global Public Health and the deputy director of the Center for Health, Identity, Behavior, and Prevention Studies at the Rutgers School of Public Health. She has expertise in HIV/AIDS, aging, resilience, vaccine sentiments, and broader LGBTQ health disparities. More specifically, her work examines resilience as it relates to biological, psychological, and social health states among older gay HIV-positive men. Dr. Krause is the founding deputy editor of *Annals of LGBTQ Public and Population Health*, a journal geared toward the health and well-being of sexual and gender diverse communities, and the deputy editor of *Behavioral Medicine*.

Nik M. Lampe
is an Assistant Professor in the Department of Mental Health Law & Policy and a Faculty Affiliate in the Louis de la Parte Florida Mental Health Institute at the University of South Florida. Their research program focuses on the behavioral health and healthcare disparities of LGBTQIA+ aging populations and diverse older adults living with dementia and their family care partners. They are also core faculty with the African American Alzheimer's Caregiver Training and Support Project 2 (ACTS2 Project), a Florida-based program that offers free skills-building and support services to Black family care partners of persons living with dementia. Dr. Lampe is currently PI of a 3-year grant from the Alzheimer's Association (AARFD-23-1145127) examining Alzheimer's disease and related dementias (ADRD) risk and protective factors among LGBTQ+ older adults in the US Southeast.

Audria LB
is a Black transfeminine filmmaker, poet, and interdisciplinary artist, currently based in Durham, North Carolina. She graduated in 2017 from the University of South Carolina, with BA degrees in Media Arts and African American Studies. Having published work in Lambda Literary Award-winning *The Black Trans Prayer Book*, they are currently a co-director on the upcoming Black Trans Prayer Book Documentary.

Ginny Natale
was an early-stage investigator focused on elucidating mechanisms between inflammatory changes, proteomics and dementia and/or cognitive decline trajectories in older adults. Her works used a pattern recognition algorithm of longitudinal cognitive data and physical health measures to detect patterns of cognitive decline indicative of probable Alzheimer's and related dementias (ADRD). She was awarded the Gerontological Society of America's Diversity

Junior Investigator Fellowship for 2020–2021. Dr. Natale was dedicated to a career as an independent investigator in the fields of Aging Epidemiology and ADRD. She was applying for a mentored NIH K01 award; her own work continues to light the path for others following in her footsteps.

Alexandra "Xan" C.H. Nowakowski
is an Associate Professor in the Geriatrics & Behavioral Sciences and Social Medicine departments at Florida State University College of Medicine. They are a medical sociologist and public health program evaluator focused on aging with chronic disease and related social justice issues. Currently they serve as lead evaluator for the Florida Asthma Program, FSU's collaborative REACH Geriatrics Workforce Enhancement Program, and the ACTS 2 training and support program for African American dementia caregivers. They also co-founded the Write Where It Hurts project on scholarship engaging lessons from lived experience of hardship and trauma, drawing on their own history with the progressive genetic disease cystic fibrosis and post-traumatic stress from domestic abuse.

Kirsten L. Ostergren Clark
is currently an Assistant Professor of Sociology and Social Work at Wilberforce University in Ohio. She graduated with her PhD in Medical Sociology from the Department of Medical Sociology at the University of Alabama at Birmingham in 2021. Her research interests are Developmental Disabilities (IDD), Masculinity and Fatherhood, and Religion and Health. She earned a Master of Social Work degree from the University of South Carolina and spent several years supervising group homes for individuals with IDD. Dr. Clark has taught sociology, psychology, and public health at the undergraduate level. She has done research work with DHS in Oklahoma and South Carolina and with Preventive Health through UAB Department of Medicine.

Manacy Pai
is an Associate Professor of Sociology at Kent State University. They have two main research interests: Social Gerontology and Medical Sociology. Their entire program of research focuses on understanding later life health. Their early studies as well as their recent and ongoing work thus center aging and older adults.

J.E. Sumerau
is an Associate Professor and the Director of Applied Sociology at the University of Tampa. They are also the author 7 novels and over a dozen short stories

published by academic presses, literary journals, and magazines including the George Garrett Fiction Prize winning coming of middle age novel *Transmission*. They are also the author of 5 nonfiction books and over 100 articles and chapters at the intersection of sexualities, gender, religion, sports, health, and violence including the examination of masculinities in society called *Violent Manhood*. For more information, please visit www.jsumerau.com

Michele Wise Wright
has championed a diverse range of health equity initiatives as the Co-Founder, Board Chair, and Senior Executive Director of the National Organization of African Americans with Cystic Fibrosis (NOAACF). With advanced degrees in engineering and public policy, she is fully committed to diversity and inclusion with a special emphasis on health equity. With NOAACF she works to ensure that racial minority communities including Black and Indigenous people are well informed of the existence, prevalence, and impact of cystic fibrosis on underrepresented communities. She led the development of The Wright Cystic Fibrosis Screening Tool© for patients and providers speaking English and/or Spanish. She also wrote, directed, and produced the award-winning short film *54 Years Late*, chronicling her husband Terry's journey to his eventual cystic fibrosis diagnosis in midlife.

Terry Gene Wright
is the Co-Founder and President of NOAACF, a 501(c)(3) organization with a mission to connect individuals with CF, help build diverse communities, and raise awareness within the African American community and beyond. He also co-founded and co-chairs the annual BIOMERGD (Blacks, Indigenous, and Other Minority Ethnicities with Rare and Genetic Diseases) Conference and led the development of a Cystic Fibrosis screening tool to help individuals self-identify symptoms that could be related to CF and doctors potentially identify individuals with CF, including individuals who are black, indigenous and people of color (BIPOC). He shares his life experiences that inspired this work in the *54 Years Late* documentary on late diagnosis of CF in African American patients and authored the award-winning children's book *Terry's Journey to CF Land* chronicling his journey.

Introduction

Alexandra "Xan" C.H. Nowakowski and J.E. Sumerau

With the publication of "Out of the Shadow: Partners Managing Illness Together" in 2017, we joined a growing chorus of other researchers, writers, and activists calling for more attention to the ways people, individually and collectively, live with and experience health and aging with chronic mental and/or physical health conditions. These efforts require people in different social and generational groups to strategically navigate visible and invisible aspects of the life course, health status, health care access or lack thereof, intergenerational interaction, and other factors that all fundamentally shape the psychological, physical, and social aspects of selfhood and the life course itself. In this volume, we have taken another step in this ongoing conversation by coordinating a collection of case studies highlighting some methods of aging invisibly as a result of specific health conditions and/or in relation to occupying specifical marginalized social locations.

With this new collection we build on our previous work utilizing case studies to illustrate significant variations and commonalities embedded within a given phenomenon. Specifically, each case study in this volume introduces, illustrates, and analyzes a form of aging invisibly while also suggesting potential avenues for improving these experiences and outcomes on multiple levels of our shared social world. Rather than attempting to summarize issues in health and aging exhaustively, the authors in this volume each provide insight into a specific case of aging invisibly through a detailed case study, experiential reflection, and/or critical review. Chapters may thus be read collectively as a broad introduction to types of aging invisibly—and health disparities—people negotiate in contemporary society. They may also be used individually as discrete learning activities for other courses and projects.

Overall, the nine cases contained in this volume take readers into the heart of significant issues faced by people growing older with chronic health conditions. The collection itself takes readers through multiple points of emphasis in health aging including but not limited to illness management, reciprocity in relationships, care work, the intersection of medical models and personal experiences, and resiliency. Chapters are also written as complete cases, which allows teachers, activists, and others in need of a solo case study to utilize any of these works as is. Finally, each reading draws from the expertise and experience specific to its authors—thus providing insights established throughout professional and personal efforts over time.

 | DOI:10.1163/9789004708136_001

We begin the following collection with an examination of how people negotiate living with Crohn's disease. Specifically, Natale and Pai outline the broader context of disabilities and diagnosis in contemporary societies as well as the existing scholarship on navigating such issues. They utilize interviews with people living with Crohn's to tease out and discuss both how people navigate the condition in daily life as well as some ways other people and health care operations specifically can better understand and respond to people with chronic illnesses. Their examination serves as both an introduction to the broader politics of chronic health conditions and an illustration of chronic illness management as an active experience.

The importance of understanding and action return in the second case study where Wise Wright and Wright discuss living with and loving people with chronic health conditions. Specifically, Wise Wright and Wright outline their own experiences with Lupus and Cystic Fibrosis respectively. They use their own relationship as a mechanism for understanding the intersection of social statuses, chronic health conditions, and romantic relationships. In so doing, they demonstrate how living and loving with chronic health conditions—as with any other details about a person—create both negative and positive situations, issues, and spaces for the active negotiation of life, love, aging, health, and societal inequalities all at once.

Next, we turn to a clinical analysis by Johnson and DiCarlo. Drawing on clinical vignettes, these scholars explore ways to combat ageism and ableism in clinical settings. Specifically, they demonstrate how these ideological biases develop and find voice throughout our social world, and impact how clinicians view patients and potential situations. With this background in mind, they then explore and discuss possible methods and theoretical frameworks for combatting these issues and creating more inclusive and respectful clinical practices. Further, their analysis focuses on how patient experiences with trauma and other negative events show up on the body, in the search for treatment, and during clinical interactions. In so doing, they call for a more nuanced and understanding approach to care work within and beyond clinical settings.

The limitations and possibilities of clinical settings also find voice in the next case wherein a transgender medical student reflects on experience in medical education. Drawing on observations before and during medical school coursework, Jones outlines the methods whereby ignorance of transgender populations and issues permeate existing medical and broader scientific and healthcare scholarship. Further, Jones illustrates how these patterns show up during interactions with medical school faculty and administrators as well as with other healthcare workers in clinical settings beyond the classroom. Finally,

Jones raises questions about the work that would need to be done to transform existing medical education and training systems.

Krause's ensuing chapter likewise explores existing medical education and training systems—focusing on experiences of older people living with HIV/AIDS. This study extends lessons from the prior chapter more broadly by examining how older people living with HIV/AIDS navigate and negotiate existing medical systems that do and do not fit their needs as an aging population. Krause calls for greater examinations of how existing protocols both do and do not work in hopes of creating more effective strategies. Further, the analysis of older people's experience of HIV/AIDS reveals the importance of paying attention to resilience in communities managing chronic health issues as well as the possibilities of revising care standards—in clinical and educational settings—based on the feedback of patient groups.

The following chapter then develops this notion of the importance of the patient as an educator for the authorities, scholars, and other members of the medical system. Specifically, working with Audria LB, Hunt reflects on the experience of growing up in the face of ongoing forms of trauma from youth into adulthood as well as some ways social statuses (i.e., race, sexuality, class, familial background, and gender) influenced these experiences. With this background in mind, Hunt and LB then explore the relationship between these factors and HIV/AIDS diagnosis as well as the powerful potential of proper diagnosis, treatment, and care during a life. These factors all combine to paint a powerful portrait of the interaction between standard of healthcare available and accessible and social statuses and locations in the outcomes of a given person facing, navigating, negotiating, and making sense of chronic conditions and other aspects of a life course.

This level of complexity comes to the forefront in Ostergren Clark's examination of fathers' experiences with children who have developmental disabilities. In this case, Ostergren Clark explores how these fathers define their parental role in relation to the chronic health conditions of their children as well as their own work in caring for adult children. Specifically, the fathers note the ways their own lives are intrinsically linked to the life course and developmental needs of their children in specific, long term, and nuanced ways. Ostergren Clark draws out insights on how such links complicate existing expectations of the life course as well as how someone else's chronic illness can impact the trajectory of others in their social world.

How any chronic condition can shift life course expectations occupies a central place in Lampe's exploration of eating disorder management. Specifically, Lampe utilizes autoethnography to examine how life course perspectives on health and aging may enhance understanding, responses to, and management strategies for disordered eating. In so doing, Lampe reviews existing research on eating disorders as a mechanism for demonstrating how different frameworks and assumptions can limit societal and scientific understanding of a given chronic condition. They then build on this insight by illustrating how patient science and lived experiences can bridge gaps in other perspectives by revealing the active processes that go into living with and managing any chronic illness in relation to existing social norms.

Patient science and autoethnographic methods likewise prove indispensable in the final case study—Nowakowski provides a review of multiple prior autoethnographic works they have utilized to extend scientific understanding of chronic illness management over the life course. In so doing, Nowakowski points to the possibilities offered by patient-science wherein the life course of a given person becomes an ongoing stream of data for analysis and consideration in the development, revision, and evaluation of scientific understanding, protocol, and process. In fact, Nowakowski demonstrates how this type of reciprocal relationship could benefit the entirety of relationships between people living with chronic conditions and health systems created to respond to such issues. Our collection of case studies closes with a call for recognizing the importance of reciprocity between research, reflection, and practice within and beyond clinical settings. We hope this inspires innovation and solidarity between people living with chronic conditions and the clinical and community professionals who support us on our unique health and aging journeys.

CHAPTER 1

"Spend Your Spoons Wisely"

Conceptualizations of Time, Energy, and Aging Invisibly with Crohn's Disease

Ginny Natale and Manacy Pai

In excess of 70 million Americans aged 50 and above live with, at least, one chronic condition (Centers for Disease Control, 2018). Moreover, an increasing proportion of persons under the age of 50 comprising a growing number of millennials are reporting, at least, one chronic ailment (Children's Health Defense, 2019; Harris Poll Survey, 2016; Transamerica Center for Health Studies, 2016). "For eight of 10 health conditions, millennials are experiencing double-digit increases in prevalence compared to what Gen Xers experienced at the same ages" (Children's Health Defense Team Report, 2019, p. 1; Blue Cross Blue Shield (BCBS) Association). Data from the National Center for Health Statistics (NCHS, 2018) in 2018 found 6.5% of adults aged 18–44 to report disability in carrying out daily activities due to a chronic disease. And yet we as a nation remain rather unprepared for a growing number of younger adults that are aging *with* chronic conditions—some that are disabling and invisible.

While the original definition of successful aging and the idea that the absence of a chronic illness or/and disability is a barometer to measure successful aging has been confronted by its many detractors (Bowling & Dieppe, 2005; Martinson & Berridge, 2015; Molton & Yorkston, 2017; Liu & Richardson, 2012; Strawbridge et al., 2002), this criterion is found in a great number of studies assessing what it means to age successfully (Depp & Jeste, 2006; Molton & Yorkston, 2017; Phelan & Larson, 2002). The unrelenting attention to the "absence" of illness in the academic literature actually mirrors the never-ending social and cultural objective of keeping separate and distinct the experiences of aging and disability from those of being young and able. And, although more recent studies have moved beyond this narrow way of defining successful aging to include the experiences of older adults with chronic illness and disability (Katz & Calasanti, 2015; Marks, 2018; Molton & Yorkston, 2017), what remains missing is research on the experience of aging among young adults living with chronic illness. In other words, we do not yet know what aging "with" a chronic and often disabling illness means for the non-elderly population. We are far less aware of the experience of aging among those Americans who instead of aging "into" disability are aging "with" it (Verbrugge & Yang, 2002).

 | DOI:10.1163/9789004708136_002

Our study fills this existing gap in the literature by assessing the process of aging with chronic illness by interviewing young adults living with Crohn's Disease, both a physically and emotionally debilitating, and often an invisible chronic condition. Data are drawn from 35 interviews with individuals living with CD, a chronic inflammatory condition of the gastrointestinal tract characterized by intermittent flare-ups of pain, weakness, fatigue, cramping, and/or diarrhea. While diet and stress may aggravate CD, they are not causally predictive of it. Recent research has suggested that genetics and/or environmental factors may contribute to the development of CD, but relatively less is known of its etiology due to genetic variability and complexity of immune responses within the gastrointestinal tract (McGovern, 2015; Park & Jeen, 2019).

1 Aging "with" Disabling Chronic Illness

Understanding the process of aging among the non-elderly population living with a chronically disabling illness is important given that it defies the social and cultural expectation of how young age and youthfulness go hand-in-hand with good health and a disability-free life. We equate chronic illness with old age, and chronic health conditions do, indeed, emerge in middle-age through later life (Wolff et al., 2002). Given the expectedness of chronic conditions in later life, older adults may be more mentally prepared for it compared to their younger counterparts (Neugarten, 1968). In fact, some research finds that being chronically ill is less stigmatizing for older as compared to younger individuals (Borawski et al., 1996; Erler & Garstecki, 2002). Compared to their younger peers, older adults with chronic illness also are more likely to secure positive verifications (Menec & Perry, 1995), which may aid in coping with the illness.

Moreover, given the prevalence of chronic illnesses in later life (Williamson & Schulz, 1995; Wolff et al., 2002), older adults may already know others in their social network with varying health conditions. While this may not erase the physical toll that a chronic illness takes, it may help older adults grapple with the stigma that is attached to several chronic illnesses. As adults, we often equate our own aging process to that of our similarly aged peers (Festinger, 1954; Staudinger, 2015; Ubel et al., 2005). The standards we set for our own aging process are shaped by these social comparisons (Stephan et al., 2013). If we think we fare better—socially, physically, and financially—than our similarly aged peers, we consequently are likely to feel more youthful than our actual chronological (i.e., biological) age (Cheng et al., 2007; Frieswijk et al., 2004). And not only are such favorable social comparisons protective of mental health (Heidrich & Ryff, 1993a, 1993b), younger age identities are associated with fewer functional limitations (Rejeski et al., 2001) and a reduced risk of mortality (Kotter-Grühn et al., 2009). For younger adults a disabling chronic illness is not only far less normative and unexpected, it also is an experience they are less exposed to in their age-matched peer groups. Social comparisons, consequently, may be more damaging to the sense of self and identity of a younger adult compared to their counterparts on the other end of the age spectrum.

Those in their 20's, 30's and 40's are expected to achieve certain socially and culturally prescribed developmental milestones and these milestones are expected to transpire by certain age and in a specific sequence (Bernsten & Ruben, 2004; Neugarten et al., 1965). People living with chronic illness and/or disability often experience major shifts in the otherwise normative life course transitions, including interrupted work, delayed marriage, and missed parenthood. Studies on the impact of chronic conditions on employment, for instance, have found that chronically ill individuals are less likely to remain employed (Reeuwijk et al., 2017; Schofield et al., 2012; Schuring et al., 2013; West et al., 2006; Van Rijn et al., 2014); and those employed are likely to feel stigmatized in the workplace (Butler & Modaff, 2016; McGonagle & Barnes-Farrell, 2014). Job loss and episodic employment histories translate into both, loss of earnings and a diminished self-worth. Plans for building a family also are likely to take a hit. Individuals with certain illnesses, for instance, are less likely to marry (DeVivo & Richards, 1996) and/or venture into parenthood given concerns of genetic spread of their condition to their offspring and/or rendering their children with the massive responsibility of caring for them in later life (LaDonna et al., 2015). Some may want to become parents but are unable to conceive given complications associated with fertility (Pebdani et al., 2014).

Given that chronic illness can not only be physically disabling but also emotionally, socially, and financially draining, it is no surprise that chronic diseases also are associated with higher prevalence of depression (Anderson et al., 2001; Chapman et al., 2005) and anxiety (Anderson et al. 2001; Chapman et al., 2005). As challenging as it is to alter one's plans for work and family transitions, equally challenging is to manage everyday symptoms of chronic illness alongside both work and family responsibilities. Altering plans, however, may be even more cumbersome for younger adults compared to their older peers given that young adulthood typically is utilized to establish oneself in terms of both, work and family. For example, for individuals hoping to excel at work or/and raise young children, pain and fatigue and the often unpredictable nature of some chronic conditions may impose limits on their life goals (Becker, 1997; Bury, 2001; Charmaz, 1991, 1999). Compared to older adults who are closer to retirement, for those in their younger years, managing chronic illness alongside both family and work responsibilities can create enormous stress. Thus, while chronic illness may cast a shadow on one's life regardless of age, being diagnosed with a disabling chronic condition can be particularly challenging for the emotional, social, and financial health of younger adults.

2 Crohn's—Invisible and Disabling Chronic Illness

Crohn's disease is a subtype of chronic inflammatory bowel disease (IBD) characterized by segments of inflammation along any portion of the digestive tract, including the mouth and/or rectum (Crohn's & Colitis Foundation of America, n.d.). Most commonly occurring between the ages of 10 and 40, a small proportion of CD cases are seen in persons in their late 50's and 60's. While there are periods of normalcy with no active symptoms, most individuals living with CD have to remain on a constant alert for a relapse of active disease known as a "flare." The symptoms during these active flare-ups include but are not limited to fluctuations in weight, abdominal cramps, nausea, vomiting, diarrhea, and fatigue. Most patients will eventually require surgery for their disease resulting from fistulas, bowel obstructions or when the anal sphincter does not function properly. Unfortunately, surgery is not curative, and patients still require ongoing medication therapy—including immunosuppressants—even after surgery to control the inflammation and induce a clinical remission (Crohn's & Colitis Foundation of America, n.d.).

Some select symptoms reported by young children are different than those observed in older persons, such as delayed growth and malnutrition (Ishige, 2019). These issues in childhood, if not treated properly, can manifest in more severe cases of CD as people age even though the disease course appears to be similar across age groups (Rosen et al., 2015). Most common clinical symptoms among the young include severe abdominal pain, diarrhea, and anemia with possible complications including fistulas, adhesions, scarring and intestinal abscesses, whereas most older adults living with CD report loss of weight, bleeding, fever, and constipation (Crohn's & Colitis Foundation of America, n.d.). Moreover, while the onset and progression of CD among the elderly tend to be much milder and stable, the opposite holds true for young adults who are diagnosed with CD (Crohn's & Colitis Foundation of America, n.d.). Understanding what it means to live and age with a disabling illness like CD is important because younger adults with this illness have significantly more number of years to have to "negotiate with and train caregivers" (Molton & Yorkston, 2017, p. 295) who also may happen to be in similar age-range (e.g., friends, spouses, co-workers). Lastly, grappling with CD may be more emotionally draining for younger individuals given that compared to their older counterparts, younger adults have fewer social and psychological resources, and coping strategies (for review, see Carstensen et al., 2003); they also are more likely than older adults to engage in self-blame (Folkman et al., 1987; Piazza et al., 2007).

In what ways, then, are young adults prepared for the social, economic and emotional challenges that accompany daily living with a chronic illness? In what ways do chronically ill young adults negotiate with and navigate through the complexities associated with their constantly evolving bodies and the restrictive values surrounding what it means to be young and old? A vast majority of existing studies do not have answers to these questions as most research related to aging and illness includes the elderly. Given that aging is an individualized process with different people aging in differing ways, at varying paces, it is only logical to assume that the pathways to successful aging also are just as distinct. Given that physiological change or functional deterioration often is associated with increasing age (Tay et al., 2019), and psychological and social aspects of aging may not necessarily parallel physiological change across the life span (Saadeh et al., 2020), we propose that certain psychological (e.g., emotional resilience) and/or social mechanisms (e.g., social support) may compensate for physiological decline and allow some individuals to age successfully, whereas others do not.

3 Methods

3.1 *Recruitment*

Online recruitment posts and in-person handouts were approved by the IRB (#16-344) prior to data collection. The first author gained access to five separate support groups by requesting to join the group and subsequently gained written permission from an administrator of the group to post recruitments for the study. The social media pages focused on social support for people living with CD. Recruitment posts were visible to all group members whereby people could voluntarily contact the researcher for more information or to schedule an interview over the telephone. The sample was predominantly female, which is not surprising considering women are more likely to volunteer in research (Smith, 2008) signaling a potential limitation recruiting from social media support groups. While both men and women use online support groups, they engage in online support for different reasons, where men were more than twice as likely to give information about their illness, while women more than twice as likely to give encouragement and social support (Wright & Schwager, 2008).

3.2 *Sample*

The first author conducted 35 semi-structured interviews with persons diagnosed with CD. Participants were recruited through snowball sampling (n = 10) and criterion sampling (n = 25) from five different support groups that communicate and meet online through social media. Snowball sampling method entails first recruiting a handful of individuals who match the criteria for inclusion in the study followed by securing recommendations from these select individuals for additional potential interviewees (Bhattacharjee, 2012; Cohen & Arieli, 2011). As such, the initial sample grows like a rolling snowball if the initial interviewees provide referrals to additional individuals to interview. Criterion sampling, which is a purposeful sampling strategy, is where all cases that meet the study criteria are selected (Palinkas et al., 2015). Consequently, individuals volunteering to participate in the study were screened for certain criteria and were not interviewed unless they were living in the United States, were between 18–55 years old and have lived with a diagnosis of CD for more than one year.

3.3 *Interviews*

Telephone interviews lasted between 45 minutes and three hours, with an average length of 90 minutes. They were primarily conducted over the telephone, due to the: (1) geographic locations of participants, who resided in 22 different states; and (2) interviewees' health restrictions. The first author obtained written consent prior to each interview through postal mail or email. The first author asked participants a series of open-ended interview questions pertaining to four life course domains, including: education, marriage, parenthood, and career. Concerns related to "aging" "acceptance," "body," "future" and being "left behind" peers as they aged were prevalent themes, and thus warranted further study.

The open-ended interview questions were used as a semi-structured guide. That said, each participant directed their own narrative, selecting the most salient experiences for discussion. The sample size was directed by the research question and analytical requirements, such as data saturation. The first author achieved theoretical saturation when continued sampling and analyzing data yielded no new themes and the four major trajectories of "education," "career," marriage," and "parenthood" were well developed. Saturation, which often is deemed as quality control in inductive data collection, as defined by Glaser and Strauss (1967, p. 61) refers to "The criterion for judging when to stop sampling the different groups pertinent to a category is the category's theoretical saturation. Saturation means that no additional data are being found whereby the sociologist can develop properties of the category. As he sees similar instances over and over again, the researcher becomes empirically confident that a category is saturated. He goes out of his way to look for groups that stretch diversity of data as far as possible, just to make certain that saturation is based on the widest possible range of data on the category."

3.4 *Analytic Framework*

We relied on Charmaz's (2014) guidelines for grounded theory where categories and themes were derived inductively to gradually obtain the data. As data collection progressed, the first author conducted analysis and interpretation of the narratives simultaneously so that emergent themes could be used to refine the interview guide and inform pending interviews. Before importing the transcripts into the qualitative analysis software Nvivo 11 (QSR International, 2015), the first author changed all identifying information about the participants. This was followed by open coding the interviews in a line-by-line process, jotting down detailed notes on the interviews, and crafting memos along the way. The first author continued to refine the codes based on an extensive review of the literature and convert the sub-codes into axial codes that supported the core construct of chronic illness experiences and aging. Axial coding in grounded theory follows the first step of open coding. Open coding entails breaking down the data into discrete or separate parts. In axial coding, we begin to pull together from these separate parts to draw the initially not-so-obvious connections between the different codes. Put simply, with axial coding, we organize the codes we develop in open coding (Allen, 2017).

These axial codes represented overreaching patterns seen throughout the data. These patterns eventually evolved into a perspective on how chronic illness impacts one's experiences with aging, time and limited energy. The first author reported the results as direct, verbatim quotations from participants, which captured key constructs emerging from the literature and were organized into two key sections. Both authors began by examining what participants described as their experiences of aging.

3.5 *Reflexivity*

The first author is a cisgender female who grew up relatively middleclass and she received a private education until she attended graduate school for her PhD in Medical Sociology. All her life she had access to the best hospitals and physicians in the US to manage the complex liver disease she was born with—known as an inborn error of metabolism. Without a proper diagnosis soon after birth, the result is sudden death. At 16, she was diagnosed with IBD, generally, and later at 18 years old was confirmed as Crohn's in the terminal ileum of her intestines. She had access to professional psychiatrists and psychotherapists to teach her healthy coping mechanisms to handle the disruptions and setbacks associated with growing up with a severe medical condition. Recently, her condition has progressed, and she was recently diagnosed with Type 2 diabetes and chronic abdominal pain at age 32. She is married with no kids and lives independently with her husband who is a data scientist. The first author identifies as disabled.

While the first author has experienced microaggressions in response to her gendered and health-related locations, she has not experienced intense discrimination at a broad systemic level due to her race ethnicity or sexuality. She occupies a relatively privileged educational, financial, racial, and sexual social locations throughout her life has likely protected her from many experiences that other people with chronic conditions may face, such as barriers to healthcare access. Yet, her standpoint also lends some insight into medical marginalization and due to being born as a 'failure to thrive' baby and was expected to never grow up to 5 feet tall, be intellectually disabled and never being able to live independently if she survived past 18 years old. The expectation for the first author's support system was merely to survive. During primary and secondary school, the first author was absent from school approximately 30 school days each year due to recurrent infections, hospitalizations, or surgeries. During her undergraduate studies, she experienced 5 years of clinical remission and was able to focus on her education. She was well-educated in medical terminology to describe her symptoms and need for medical attention in specific ways that physicians understand. She used this familiarity with medical terminology and her own lived experiences with chronic illness to aid the interviews and probes to build rapport with her respondents. Her intimate experiences with chronic illness and the US healthcare system as a patient allowed deeper interpretation of the data. It also allowed participants to freely discuss medical terms, medications, side effects and surgeries without having to explain terms to her during the interview. she disclosed her diagnosis of CD with participants before the interview started. The participants told her repeatedly how good it feels to talk to some that really understand what it's like. By disclosing her disease as part of the research design, participants felt comfortable sharing more private information compared to another researcher that is not chronically ill. "You get it" or "I'm sure you know what that feels like" were common phrases that kept repeating.

Given the influences of the researcher on data collection, reciprocity was an important aspect of the research design as the first author was concerned about the potential power imbalance between researcher and interviewee. Beginning in the design of the study and throughout data collection, the first author wrote weekly reflective memos to be reflexive about the study. At the end of each interview, each respondent had the opportunity to ask the researcher open-ended questions. The first author was cognizant of the expectation that interviewees had for the study findings and reminded each participant that the purpose of the study was not to providing a cure or re-diagnosis.

The second author was not involved in any aspect of the data collection and as such carried no influence on it. Based on her expertise in the areas of aging and health, the contribution of the second author included the crafting and revising of this manuscript.

4 Results

The majority of the participants were high-school graduates, married, employed and parents. Respondents had a wide range of educational levels, work and occupational statuses (Table 1.1). On average, participants were 37 years of age at the time of interview. The average time since diagnosis was 17 years and ranged from 3 to 34 years. Many worked full-time outside of the home and some held advanced or graduate degrees. Most have had surgery in relation to CD in the past (63%). The sample in our study is comparable to the proportion of individuals living with CD in the US. Only N = 3 were diagnosed before 18 years old. The average age range of a CD diagnosis in the US is 15–35 (Feuerstein & Cheifetz, 2017).

Of the 35 participants interviewed, three-quarters specifically expressed worries about the future and aging specifically related to physical limitations of having CD. The other 25% expressed feelings about learning to accept the diagnosis and 'moving forward' with their life course as they age. All participants described the difficulties of fatigue and energy limitations.

5 Theme 1: Planning for the Future Is Limited to 24 Hours

All participant plans for the future were limited to 24 hours—a direct consequence of functional limitations of relapsing-remitting disease. For instance, Molly, a 28-year-old nanny and college student, explained that she needs to tackle challenges that come her way day-by-day. In her words,

> I think I'm relatively you know, I have come to terms with it. Have my freak out moments every now and then but I mean you sort of have to take it, same by saying and day by day. Just hope that at some point, they come out with a cure for it, in your lifetime.

TABLE 1.1 Participant work status and occupation (n = 35)

Name[a]	Age	Work status	Occupation	Education
Aaliyah	27	Full-time	General manager	Some college
Addison	27	Full-time	Academic advisor	Graduate/professional degree
Adriana	28	Disability	Neuroscientist	Graduate/professional degree
Alexa	40	Full-time	University professor	Graduate/professional degree
Andrea	25	Full-time	Music teacher	Graduate/professional degree
Annabelle	24	Full-time	Secretary	Bachelors
Brittany	27	Full-time	Medical assistant	High school
Brooklyn	46	Disability	Accountant IT	Bachelors
Charlie	35	Part-time	Gas station clerk	Some college
Cindy	39	Full-time	Finance claims	Associates
Daniel	37	Full-time	Attorney	Graduate/professional degree
Derek	34	Full-time	Pharmacy technician	Associates
Diana	51	Part-time	Cashier	High school
Eva	26	Part-time	Photographer	Bachelors
Faith	29	Stay-at-home	Middle school teacher	Bachelors
Farah	34	Stay-at-home	Online translator	Graduate/professional degree
Frank	50	Full-time	Factory worker	Bachelors
Gary	44	Disability	General manager	Some college
Grace	45	Full-time	TV producer	Bachelors
Hannah	39	Disability	Retail clerk	Bachelors
Katelyn	46	Disability	Radio producer	Graduate/professional degree
Katherine	42	Part-time	Church secretary	Bachelors
Katie	41	Part-time	Charity fundraiser	High school
Kylie	46	Full-time	University professor	Graduate/professional degree
Lily	25	Full-time	Registration secretary	Bachelors
Madeline	52	Disability	Supervisor teacher	Graduate/professional degree
Mazen	23	Full-time	Model	Some college
Melissa	46	Part-time	Psychologist	Bachelors
Molly	28	Full-time	Nanny & student	Bachelors
Natalie	28	Full-time	Store clerk	Some college
Savannah	51	Full-time	Factory worker	Bachelors
Seth	25	Full-time	Occupational therapist	Graduate/professional degree
Suzie	45	Full-time	Scholarship coordinator	Bachelors
Wesley	54	Full-time	IT technician	Associates
Zach	31	Disability	Home inspector	Bachelors

a All names referenced are fictitious.

Her excerpt juxtaposes the very real physical limitations of CD to 24 hours and contrasts it with hopes for the future cure for the disease—hopefully in her lifetime. Preparing for the future is always contrasted with the long-term plan for their life course. For example, Daniel, a 37-year old attorney, explains the mental mapping he attempts to coordinate for the next 30 years, but yet is prepared for things not to go as planned. He says,

> So, I haven't exactly mastered [it] out on paper, but I have taken my mind through some of those scenarios in order if we can ever prepare for that, because you don't know when it's going to happen, or if it's going to happen. But at least to prepare my mind for the possibility that something might not go as planned in the next 30 years and I might have a changed track.

While he is mapping out his future, he also simultaneously prepares to be derailed if CD results in increasing disability. Indeed, planning for the future was a key topic of most narratives. Yet, plans for the future are always qualified by what can be accomplished within one 24-hour cycle. Other participants think about death when thinking about planning for the future. Overwhelmingly, the narratives portray death as an everyday threat. Adriana, 28, described how her plans of the future differ from her peers.

> I think I think about it more than they do. I mean I have had 5 near deaths experiences and 3 of them in the last calendar year. I think more than anyone I am realistic about the fact that, yes, this disease could kill me and yes this disease does kill people and clearly I've had all kinds of different complications with it, and I do not have any sort of normal Crohn's disease.

Her narrative implies that she herself is not normal because her course of CD is different from others' experiences. So, planning for the future really is limited to the most immediate present—i.e., in terms of later in the same day or at most, the following one. The limits that a physically and emotionally unraveling illness places on people's ability to plan for the future is what separates those aging "with" disability from their peers who age "into" disability. While those aging into disability prepare for the distant future and then alter plans if health conditions emerge, those aging with disability are forced to alter plans every day in order to meet plans made for the very immediate future. Even in times of remission, flares of CD can happen, making remission a highly stressful time of monitoring symptoms daily. The daily monitoring of signs and symptoms marks the 24-hour window with worry that another flare of illness is coming soon. As Addison, 27 and full-time General Manager, described the worry that accompanies the daily threat of a flare of symptoms, saying:

> It was more nerve wrecking being in a flare because I was always waiting for the bomb to drop and I was always like thinking like oh! Like today's the day that my flare's going to come back.
>
> I think, even though I always had that fear, I also knew like you don't know how many good days before another bad day so enjoy it while it lasts type of thing. Now that I'm with the bag, it's not as nerve wrecking, it's just now anytime that something feels awful because like if I feel like I'm starting to get an abscess, I like obsessed about it and I'm like oh my God! This is an abscess, is it an ingrown hair, or is it my imagination like all together.
>
> I think that remission is enjoyable if you just take it day by day, because like again, with auto-immune diseases, you are never how long it's going to last. I've done a pretty good job with being in remission and I've learned the hard way that the minute you start having signs and symptoms, you don't push off going to the doctor you call them right away.

Even in remission, planning for the future is limited to the present. What if today is the day CD flares again? What if today is the end of remission? Imagining the future and planning ahead often is predicated on the normativeness of the life course. Lives transpire within the realm of certain social and cultural life scripts (Pecchioni, 2012) that are in place to guide both our expectations for the future and plans for it. And these scripts are not for individuals per se but societies at large and as such, they provide a may for what's to follow across the life course (Pecchioni, 2012). However, these plans are subject to constant change when aging "with" a disability. Later in her narrative, Addison stated that she had no plans when in a flare, but this had changed, stating,

> Now that I'm healthier, I definitely think about it more. When I was sick, I could care less. I was like let me just get through the next day. So, it's definitely something that the healthier I am, the more I think about.

In Addison's narrative, her plans depend on her physical health. Now that she is not "sick" –an all-encompassing state—she can plan a normative life course. One expectation that we have is that we are going to live a long and healthy life. And, as such, we have the freedom to plan for high school and college graduations, a career, a home with a white picket fence, marriage, and parenthood. However, the normativeness of the idealized life course is interrupted and even disrupted when we are faced with the otherwise unexpected negative life events. For people with CD and limited energy, choosing which negative life event to focus on necessitates prioritization. Madeline, the 52-year-old lady currently on disability and a former teacher "picks battles" and prioritizes very carefully "what really matters" to her—so that she can focus her limited energy on the most essential activity. This leads us to the subtheme of limiting and prioritizing activities.

5.1 *Subtheme 1: Limiting and Prioritizing Activities*

Limiting and prioritizing activities were essential means to maintaining successful aging for people living with an invisible chronic illness in our study. Melissa, a 46-year-old psychologist, explains how her bodily sensations limit her activities and force her to prioritize what really matters. She describes a 'process' of learning what her bodily limits are and how to respond in a way that does not threaten her survival. She describes the 3-year process for her accepting her diagnosis and new lifestyle with a disability.

> So, but the process basically was, you know, my body can't handle this and so, I need to do what's best for my body or I could lose it, I could die basically. The rational part of me accepted that. The rational part of me is like, "Well, yes, that makes total sense and it's for the best that you never had children because."

She denotes the difference between her rational and emotional thoughts. Logically, she knows scaling back her activities is better for her health, and yet she still longs to be able to do all of the activities she used to do before her diagnosis. Like the other narratives in this theme, her activities and plans are limited to a 24-hour window. Part of that 24 hours need to include rest and recuperation. Eva, a 26-year-old photographer, laments similarly that she has a hard time planning for things beyond the 24 hours, because what she does today impacts what she is able to do tomorrow and the day after. She had to stay behind as her college peers moved to Los Angeles to pursue their fine arts careers, while she stayed in her hometown to do private photography—an activity where she can manage her hours flexibly. She states,

> So, for me that was a big decision that I had to make, like staying behind… Yeah, I uh have a hard time, I have a hard time thinking individually, because every day impacts the next day. So, that's a big issue with friends that trying to plan. Like things in the future, and I'm like well I mean we can, but I have no idea what I will feel like that day. If I'll be able to do it but.

Others elaborated on how living with a chronic illness forced them to simplify their daily lives, focus on themselves and put off things for later. Frank, a 50-year-old factory laborer explained,

> That's sometimes you just have simplified things. Not have things so complicated, simplified things, keep things basic, you are forgetting it's still a funk, don't try and do 100 different things, just break down, and is this important, is this not important, can this be put off later, and just focus on you.

Similarly, Brooklyn, a 46-year-old accountant, replied that she only does the 'minimal' things for close family and friends to conserve her efforts. She said,

> Basically, only minimal or what I need to do for close family and friends. Most of my energy now is trying to figure out who can help me, and who is going to help me in doctor's way. Just finding doctors and people that actually are more wanting to help you, and not just kind of push you off on the back burner.

Addison, a 27-year-old academic advisor, also noted how important close family were in helping her cope with her illness, surgeries and diagnosis as the "darkest" moments in her life. She notes a disconnect between her relationships with her friends compared to the close emotional connectedness of her family. As such, she also prioritizes close family relationships. She noted,

> I think my friends are still at that point where it doesn't, like they don't necessarily, they see their family, but they don't make them a priority, and for me, I was like no, my family got me [through] some of the darkest times of my life. Like I make the time [for] family.

Findings from our study are reminiscent of Carstensen's (1992, 1999, 2006) socioemotional selectivity theory (SST). SST posits that "humans become increasingly selective in their goals based on their placement in the life span for the purpose of maximizing life satisfaction" (Sullivan-Singh et al., 2015, p. 2). SST, which was primarily conceived keeping in mind older adults, posits that when life appears to be limited or end of life seems proximate, older adults start to trim all the non-essential goals and social networks and prioritize instead those aspirations and relationships that they deem vital to their most immediate emotional well-being. Given that younger adults expect a prolonged life span, they often plan for a future they deem more distant. They often prioritize future investments, including planning careers and developing social networks and relationships that they expect to pay off in their later years. In contrast, older adults who "perceive their time to be limited prioritize the present with the goal of maximizing emotional gratification in the present moment" (Sullivan-Singh et al., 2015, p. 2). Life span of the participants in our study, however, is not limited; rather despite the everyday challenges they are faced with, these individuals can expect to live long and grow into old age like their counterparts without CD. Findings from our study, as such, extends the SST to include even those individuals who are diagnosed and living with an illness that does not include a limited life span with a proximate end of life. It is reasonable to assume then that the age disparity in goal selection may have less to do with age per se and more to do with restrictions on the present time. Participants in our study often comment on how, despite knowing that death is not impending, they feel like their bodies are withering away and reeling out of their control.

As participants reflect on aging, they note that little things do not bother them as much as they used to when they were younger. Cindy, a 39-year-old finance claims accountant, notes that now, at nearly 40, she cannot take big trips or plan big events that take a lot of commitment. Instead, she focuses on things that matter (i.e., "little things") like doing homework after school with her two daughters. She said,

> You know it can't be the big trips of big events or anything else. It's just all little things now. As you get older, you learn that too though. Some of that comes with age.

These findings suggest that there are few other experiences in life that clarify one's values, goals, and priorities like a chronic ailment. Living with CD is like working on a never-ending, unsolvable puzzle. You think you have all the pieces of it on the good days and good weeks and then the puzzle shifts, there are new pieces thrown into the mix, some old ones disappear, and you may have to start back again. The things that mattered at first—such as applying for a higher paying job or a promotion, planning a trip or a neighborhood get-together—all of a sudden matter a whole lot less. Instead, our findings reveal that those living with the unpredictability of CD start to focus on the most immediate of their goals and prioritize family and friends that matter most.

5.2 *Subtheme 2: Subjective Age*

Notably as participants reflected on their age and getting older, many noted that they feel older than their chronological age. Subjective aging is a comparative process contrasting how individuals feel in their body versus their chronological age. Brittany, a 26-year-old medical assistant, said how scared she is reflecting on her subjective age. She noted,

> Yeah, I have and it's really scary. Just because like if I feel 45 at 26, I can't imagine what I'm going to feel like at 45.

Brittany estimates her subjective age older than her chronological age which has been linked to physical health and cognitive decline and dementia (Kwak et al., 2018). Similarly, Lily, a 27-year-old receptionist, noted her subjective age, saying,

> But yeah, it's like I think about the fact that, it's probably not going to go backwards. I'm not going to turn 27, and all-over sudden feel 27 and relate to other 27-year old's the same way. So, I mean just something you have to get used to. My friends call me really old soul, and that I'm the mum of the friend group.

The older age identity among chronically ill young adults is not a surprise given that this finding has emerged in many studies on illness and age identity. What is troubling is that extensive research shows that feeling older than one's chronological age (i.e., an older age identity) is associated with a myriad of health troubles, as measured by anxiety and depression (Keyes & Westerhof, 2012), irregular sleep patterns (Stephan, Sutin, Luchetti, & Terracciano, 2017), incident hospitalization (Stephan, Sutin, & Terracciano, 2016), cognitive health difficulties, including higher risk of dementia (Stephan et al., 2016), and other chronic health conditions (Demakakos et al., 2007). Youthful age identities, alternatively, are accompanied by a higher sense of self-worth (Stephan et al., 2011), which protects against physical decline (Rejeski et al., 2001) and reduces the risk of mortality (Kotter-Grühn et al., 2009).

6 Theme 2: Saving Spoons and Quantifying Energy

The second most prominent theme that emerged from participants' narratives to explain aging invisibly with a chronic illness was quantifying energy into 'spoons,' objective measurements of their energy limitations. Madeline, a 52-year-old woman currently on disability and a former teacher explains:

> I mean everything is planned out, you have to think about it because you've got to be prepared for any kind of flares. Your whole life is always on

> autopilot of, "Well, okay, what can I do today? What I'm I capable of doing later?" It's really the same theory, it's like how many hours do you want me to rest before I could do X, Y, Z. Then I can't plan to do anything after work, because I know that I have to have down time to recuperate. So, yeah, I got to pick my battles and my options now very carefully about what really matters to me. So, that I can exert the energy in all of the right places.

Madeline's plans after work are limited because a significant portion of her day is dedicated to rest and recuperation from the wear and tear the day has done to her body. This narrative relates to the spoon theory, a popular vernacular by Christine Miserandino (2003) describing the limited energy a person with a chronic illness has in spoons (a second theme discussed later. Rest is necessary to recover spoons spent on everyday tasks like getting out of bed, taking a shower, driving to work, etc. Every person has a set number of spoons they can spend. Once the spoons are spent for the day, the person cannot perform more activities without rest.

Similarly, Melissa, a 46-year old psychologist, noted the life lessons having CD has taught her—namely to conserve her energy for things that are really important. She saves her spoons to be able to go to events that are important to her, asking herself if this particular activity is worth spending spoons on now if she knows she won't have spoons for tomorrow. She explained,

> I think the Crohn's helped teach me, you know, as my boyfriend would tell me, spend your spoons wisely, you know about the spoons theory, right? Yeah, and so, you know, the idea of, this, is it really going to matter in 100 years if you get an A on that test or you do XY or Z, probably not. So, don't expand any spoons over that. But prior to the crohn's, yeah, I expanded a lot of spoons on really type A kind of stuff, you know.

Similarly, Madeline, a 52-year-old former teacher now on disability relief, noted that she saved her spoons for two days to be able to see her granddaughter on Martin Luther King Jr. Day. She explained,

> So, I like went to January the Martin Luther King Day, I saved up some energy all weekend, so that I could go with my grandbaby. So, yeah, I got to pick my battles and my options now very carefully about what really matters to me. So, that I can exert the energy in all of the right places.

Notably, she said she prioritizes where to spend her spoons 'in all the right places' which relates to the previous subthemes above of prioritizing activities and limiting social interactions to close family connected to the SST theory. Madeline clearly trims her social network to focus her energy on a few special tasks and relationships.

Many participants noted their use of this strategy in planning activities that do not take up too many spoons, like attending college classes online, rather than face-to-face. For Aaliyah, a 27-year-old General Manager of a restaurant, she condensed her activities, so she was able to keep up her attendance without sacrificing her health and well-being. She said,

> Honestly it one of those where I avoided it in person classes. I did a lot of online classes. I tried to like condense my classes into like as fewer days as possible so that way, for instance all my classes were on Monday or Wednesday. So that way there was less of a chance of missing class or it's like it's only one day, I can force myself to deal with one day. So, I guess there was less energy spent.

In many ways, those with CD are forced into becoming more practical and less emotional with their time. Understanding that while life is not limited, individuals with CD come to understand that their days consist of limited units of energy, "spoons" as many refer to them. As such, unlike most humans who do not conscientiously think about the number of things they can do any given day within the context of their energies, those with CD literally calculate in their mind what tasks need to be limited today in order to ensure being able to get through the activities tomorrow. It is all about the small, attainable jobs and tasks that not only improve self-confidence but also preserve the "spoons" for the more pressing, inevitable tasks of tomorrow.

Needless to say, though, there are some that describe the constant tension of choosing which activities to pursue and spend spoons on. Aaliyah continued,

> But at the same time, it really does affect what I do. So, it's like constantly a push-pull situation and trying to pick and choose like what I do one day to that affects the next few days et cetera.

Other participants had a grimmer outlook on how many spoons are available to them to use. Gary, a 44-year-old former general manager currently on disability relief, described it as a non-choice when he said,

> Yes, yeah, I have no other option now, because I can't even do anything if I don't rest. Like right now I've been resting, take my meds resting. Then

> now I get dressed and then I go get, drive to town and take my grandbaby and do a couple of errands, and then I have to come home and rest.

6.1 *Subtheme 1: Physiological/Functional Limitations and Aging Bodies*

Related to this overarching theme, is a related sub-theme of realizing physiological and functional limitations of their aging bodies with a chronic illness. Notably most participants described in their narratives a detachment from their bodies and the likelihood of progressive disability as they age. Grace, a 45-year-old television producer, said,

> I think about my body as long as I have my mind and I can function and do the things I want to do, yes. I can't, I'm not going to be afraid of it, I'm not going to be afraid of my future, I refuse. If I can't get through that I did now, I can't get through whatever comes up and if I can still think and I can still have a mind and I have some way to communicate, the way I feel or what I'm thinking, I'll be okay.

Participants like Grace clearly deemed physical health and their body's ability to function independent important; however, they also felt the need to distinguish between their body and their mind. Also, while Grace described her body as a separate entity that she does not fear, findings also suggest that unlike their so-called "healthy and able" counterparts, those with CD are very aware of their bodies. They allow their bodies to talk to them, listen very carefully to what they have to articulate, pay heed to what they need. Unlike most young adults who dictate to their bodies their wishes, participants living with CD strive to obey the wishes of their constantly unpredictable and evolving bodies. Attending to their bodies is important, they say, because if you do not pay attention to what your body is telling you today, you may not have a body that cooperates much with you tomorrow or the day after.

Grace remains hopeful as long as she is cognitively healthy and still has her mind to think and feel emotions. As long as she can communicate with others and the outside world, she is able to cope with the additional challenges attached to aging with a chronic illness. Physical limitations were measured not only in number of spoons available to spend, but also "good days" versus "bad days." As highlighted in one autoethnography of chronic illness, patience plays a critical role in everyday illness experience (Nowakowski, 2016), as it may develop into a powerful psychological resource in the never-ending battle against a debilitating chronic condition. For Diana, a 51-year-old part-time cashier, she defines good days are those where she can do simple chores around the house and go out for a trip to the mall. Good days are when she wants to take advantage of less symptoms and less pain, so she enjoys doing mundane tasks many people take for granted. She said,

> Yeah, I have to be really careful with my energy. Because if I have a really good day, I will just like yesterday I went to the mall, and I worked and I just did some other things, and it was too much, but I had a good day. I think while I have a good day, well get as much as I can get done, I have to change that thinking very soon. Because I'm having a good day, maybe wash the dishes in the kitchen, wash the pots and pans for the kitchen and I go to the mall.

Good days are distinguished by busy work and manual chores—chores that take energy. When participants have good days, or days without pain, they prefer to be physically active and social. In addition to the good days, participants also noted how CD accelerated their body's aging. Katherine, 42-year-old mother of four young children. She works part-time the secretary of the local church, where her husband is a second-generation pastor. In her narrative below, she details how her body has changed from CD,

> I know, it kind of is. But I can't say they messed me up. There are so many other people that have had worst issue, I can't say they messed me up. It's just a very slow process. Okay so, along this stretch there [points to belly], after we did the original [intestinal] bulge thing, I started to get into pain. My neck started to get horrendously out of alignment, and I kind of started falling apart, does that make sense? And of course, I'm older and so my core is probably mush.

Like Katherine, Eva noticed her body "falling apart" too, saying, "Just get my health back together, because for four years up until on August, I was the healthiest I've ever been. Since August I've sort fallen way off where I get inflammation. So, my main priority is to get back to that place. The imagery of participants describing their bodies as they age as "falling apart" was very common. Participants grapple with bodies that fail them and are in pain everyday, like Aaliyah. She stated,

> Because I feel like I've achieved a lot in my life for having been in pain every day. Like I'm really proud of where I am and how much I get done every day with being in pain every day…Like the thing that really irritates me is that people don't realize that it affects your joints, it affects your

> eyes, it affects your mouth, it affects your skin, it affects your mental well-being. The fact that people don't realize that everything that it entails.

Not only does CD impact one's physical health, it also can diminish participants' body image and how they relate to their self through their bodies. Molly, a 28-year-old young lady who works as a part-time nanny and student, described her connection with her body after living with CD for 10 years, saying

> My body image is I think my body image is not okay. For me when I look at myself in the mirror I'm not happy and for me when I'm around people I'm very self-conscious about things and my belly not sticking out. I'm very conscious of how people perceive me and how people are looking at I feel like everyone's just staring at me when probably that's not the case at all. I just feel like Crohn's has taken so much from me and the medication have taken so much from me that I feel like I can't get myself back.

As Turner (1984, p. 1) said, "There is an obvious and prominent fact about human beings: They have bodies, and they *are* bodies. More lucidly, human beings are embodied, just as they are enselved." Molly's experience with her illness and the resulting bodily changes point exactly to this fact that notions of self and identity are inextricably linked to the notions we hold of our body, our perceptions of how we appear to and are evaluated by others (Gecas, 1989). As Molly and others age with disability, they age within their embodied selves—weaving a complex narrative of the body, selves and aging "with" a disabling chronic condition.

7 Discussion

The leading cause of death has shifted from infectious to chronic non-communicable diseases (World Health Organization, 2015). We also have witnessed enormous medical and technological advancements over the past half century. As such, an increasing number of people with chronic medical disabilities today are living longer and into old age (Huygens et al., 2016; Leray et al., 2016; Strauss et al., 2006; World Health Organization, 2015). For instance, while still lower compared to the general population, the life expectancy for people with degenerative chronic conditions, such as relapsing-remitting multiple sclerosis (RRMS) continues to increase over time (Marrie et al., 2010; Scalfari et al., 2013). Similarly, those with conditions, such as spinal cord injury (DeVivo & Chen, 2011; Strauss et al., 2006) can expect to live lot longer than their peers in the previous generation (DeVivo & Chen, 2011; Noonan et al., 2012; Strauss & Day, 2007).

While individuals with such chronic illnesses are said to age "with" disability, their counterparts without chronic conditions age "into" it (Verbrugge & Yang, 2002). Our findings reveal the experience of aging "with" a disability as our respondents who are living with CD limit their planning to the proximate future of 24 hours and prioritize activities, events, and people that matter most "now" as opposed to investing in distant goals and relationships they deem are out of reach. We also find that while participants in our study have learned to cope with the erratic nature of their disease, the constant ups and downs associated with CD and the weathering of the body via toxic stress (Geronimus, 1992) and chronic medical gaze of their body-mind (Foucault, 1973, 1980) they endure render them feeling older than they actually are. Indeed, weathering of the body here has less to do with the otherwise normative aging process and more to do with the enduring of the deluge of insults to the body of those living with CD. As Brittany, 27, noted, "Just because like if I feel 45 at 26, I can't imagine what I'm going to feel like at 45." Some, however, reckon that while their body may endure the wear and tear and "fall apart" (Katherine, 42), their mind still is intact and the cognitive acuity they still possess is what matters most for their sense of self. As Grace, 45, reflected, "I can still have a mind and I have some way to communicate, the way I feel or what I'm thinking, I'll be okay."

These findings, we argue, are important insights into the process of aging for those who live and age "with" a chronic illness as their everyday lives are immersed in managing the varying whims of that illness. What makes Crohn's particularly difficult is the unpredictable, often exacerbating-relapsing nature of the disease (Torres et al., 2017). While coping with the erratic nature of the disease is frustrating, respondents in our study have learned how to cope with the unexpected by disengaging from certain activities, curtailing the level of involvement in others, and delegating responsibilities on to others that once were carried out by them. Many commented that the value of disengaging from unrealistic tasks and limiting oneself to small, attainable goals is that the latter resulted in a greater perceived self-adequacy and improved self-morale. For instance, Grace said doing chores improved her mood on a 'good day,' saying "maybe wash the dishes in the kitchen, wash the pots and pans for the kitchen." Good days, in our study, are distinguished by physical activity, usually small tasks, busy work and manual chores.

While on one hand, living with CD limits planning for the future, on the other hand, it forces individuals living with CD daily to look closely at things that matter most in the present. As such, our findings reveal that be it decisions related to school (Aaliyah, 27), work (Addison, 27), or family (Cindy, 39

& Brooklyn, 46), our respondents who are living with CD are coping with this illness by prioritizing what is most meaningful to them in their present time. For instance, Aaliyah, a full-time General Manager, decided to take all of her classes condensed to two days per week to limit the energy spent traveling and studying every day. Meanwhile, Addison, an Academic Advisor, made decisions to pursue an academic office job advising students which allowed her to manage her symptoms better with a predictable schedule. Both Cindy and Brooklyn decided their family is their priority and made decisions according to their children's needs as well as their physical health needs. As Brooklyn, on disability from accounting, stated her energy is very limited, focused on family, and "Most of my energy now is trying to figure out who can help me, and who is going to help me in doctor's way." While as most humans, these individuals too would like to plan for the future, they have found the value in tending to the present, as Madeline, 52, said, "Well, okay, what can I do today?"

When time is perceived to be limited or finite—either because of aging or illness—individuals turn attention to more proximate and tangible goals instead of investing in plans with distant dividends (Fredrickson & Carstensen, 1990; Fung et al., 1999). Proponents of the socioemotional selectivity theory (Carstensen et al., 1999) suggest that the perception of limited time leads to preferences for goals, plans, and activities that provide instantaneous and practical value over ones with a long-term worth. Our findings, however, showcase that even when the future is not finite, the everyday complications associated with a chronic disease force people to forgo plans for the future, like Cindy, 39, and instead prioritize on more immediate goals with immediate payoffs, like completing homework assignments with her two girls aged 9 and 11. It is not the finite time but the finite number of energies or "spoons" that are available on any given day that dictates what is planned for the foreseeable future of the 24 hours. Spoons are a limited resource that is not to be wasted. Participants were very careful noting how they spent each spoon. As Melissa, 46, noted the mental calculation saying, "is it really going to matter in 100 years if you get an A on that test or you do XY or Z, probably not. So, don't expand any spoons over that."

The finding of finite energies and its relevance to the management of one's everyday lives is reminiscent of the Spoon Theory, developed by Christine Miserandino in 2003. Miserandino who has lupus, describes the events of a typical day (e.g., showering, dressing, eating, working, socializing) and taking away 1 or more spoons per activity. When the spoons are spent, the day's activities are over. While it is possible to exceed one's daily limit, doing so means borrowing from the future, which may mean having left with fewer spoons for the following day. Melissa, a 46-year-old psychologist working part-time, used to "waste" spoons on "Type A stuff" and stress over inconsequential things that, now having CD, are not worth spending spoons on. CD, she asserts has "taught" her lessons in life about prioritizing and "spending spoons wisely." Others like Madeline, 52, save their spoons for special events to see close family members. For Madeline, currently on disability from full-time teaching, she knows that going to see her granddaughter will require all of her saved up spoons but forging that meaningful relationship with her granddaughter is worth the exhaustion of resources.

This is not surprising given that Crohn's is highly unpredictable; and, the unpredictability of Crohn's is what adds ambiguity about the future, which can be distinct from many other chronic conditions that lay out a more predictable course of illness (Wilkinson & Nair, 2013). Findings from our study point out to the difficulty faced by respondents in understanding, planning, and preparing for all of the expected and unexpected symptoms of their illness. Moreover, even the symptoms a person comes to expect having lived with Crohn's may be more or less severe during each flare-up—not to mention the lack of insight into the timing of a flare-up. For instance, Addison, 27, noted the uncertainty saying, "I was always waiting for the bomb to drop and I was always like thinking like oh! Like today's the day that my flare's going to come back."

What evokes anxiety and prevents long-term planning is the fear of the unknown. Despite research on medical facets of Crohn's and the stigma associated with symptoms of CD (e.g., irritable bowel, rectal bleeding), attention to how those living with this condition cope with it remains missing. For instance, we know little of the everyday stressors and strategies deployed by those living and coping with this condition. Research on several other chronic illnesses, such as cancer and MS, indicates the strain that these illnesses inflict upon individuals. The personal, social, and psychological consequences of Crohn's, however, remain largely unexplored.

We speculate that the lack of attention given to everyday coping with Crohn's is reflective of the invisibility associated with this condition. Unlike several chronic illnesses where symptoms are obvious, symptoms of Crohn's are not always visible. Symptoms, such as gastrointestinal distress, muscle weakness, chronic fatigue or pain can disrupt a person's everyday activity, but these symptoms do not make the distress experienced by that person obvious to the observers. While there are clear advantages to the invisibility of the symptoms, disadvantages associated with it also are plenty. Cultural representations of CD reduce this condition to symptoms of bowel control at the expense of ignoring the gravely disruptive nature of this illness, which makes coping with it an everyday challenge. Incomplete representations of CD perpetuates the misconception that it is just a "pooping disease," as Andrea (25) and Charlie (35) stated in their interviews in response to media depictions of CD in popular pharmaceutical advertisements.

Our findings also show that individuals living with Crohn's are constantly learning about their illness and consequently, their bodies. They do not deny their illness; instead, they listen keenly to what their bodies are telling them. For instance, Cindy, a 49-year-old financial claims associate, said "So, I know my body inside and out and If I'm telling somebody I feel certain way, then because I still have that thing with my ex-husband. I have to do all the questions in my head, am I really feeling like this or what but yeah. My body is not lying to me. That's pretty much it." Instead of dictating to their bodies, those living with Crohn's learn to pay close attention to the everyday musings of their bodies as Addison, 27 said, "I've learned the hard way that the minute you start having signs and symptoms, you don't push off going to the doctor you call them right away." And, in doing so, they both cope and accept the realities of their illness. Acceptance, we argue, is one way of coping because it allows an individual to redefine and cognitively reinterpret their bodies and in turn, their sense of self. One way of coping with their illness and changing bodies is to understand that while the body and mind are connected, they also are separate entities. Although the bodies may betray, one participant commented on how it is the mind that maintains a sense of sanity.

Having said that, the intimate attention to their constantly evolving body, including the incessant wear and tear of it has rendered a few of our participants feeling significantly older than their actual age. Clarke and Korotchenko (2011, p. 1) in their work on aging and the body point out that "it is in and through our bodies that we most immediately experience the social and physical realities of growing older. Whether it is the development of wrinkles, grey hair, or age spots, the onset of health conditions such as arthritis, osteoporosis, or prostate cancer, or the sting of ageism in our social interactions, all of our experiences of aging are invariably embodied." Put simply, the aging bodies express themselves through a variety of symptoms, such as lack of sleep, soreness, stiff joints, and inflexible muscles. And, through these symptoms these bodies set limits to what we can plan for or handle on any given day. Older adults, for this reason, are acutely aware of their changing bodies as their bodies report to them every day. Similarly, young adults with CD also are in constant and intimate contact with their bodies which makes the process of aging a more proximate than distant experience. It is not unexpectedly then that some of our respondents report feeling older than their actual chronological age. An older subjective age identity also is a result of experiencing a chronic illness, which while older adults perceive to be an inevitable consequence of growing old (Sanders et al., 2002), younger adults may find it trickier to normalize. While most older people report feeling younger than their chronological or biological age (Cleaver & Muller, 2002; Oberg & Tornstam, 2001), dwindling health and uncooperative bodies often result in older age identities (Barrett, 2003; Hubley & Russell, 2009).

7.1 *Limitations and Future Directions*

First, while geographical dispersion in terms of participants is a definite strength in that it allows for maximization in geographical diversity, it also introduces confounding elements to the data that inductive nature of our study precludes us from controlling for. Second, we are unable to control for several other conceptually relevant factors, such as disease trajectory. It is possible that with time, individuals with chronic illness garner more stable forms of support and psychosocial resources in addition to better emotional and practical coping strategies as they continue to grapple with the disruptions they are faced with due to their illness. Third, we lack demographic diversity in our sample. That is, we do not have a racially and ethnically diverse sample and the gender distribution also is not adequate enough to draw any gender-based conclusions related to how younger adults live, cope, and age with Crohn's.

Assessing race and gender variations in aging with CD is important in the light of existing findings on race and gender variations in coping with other chronic illnesses. Compared to their white peers, Black Americans with diabetes, for instance, report on an average more mental distress (Li et al., 2008). Similarly, women with cancer (Baider et al., 1989; Linden et al., 2012), type 2 diabetes (Demmer et al., 2016), and coronary heart disease (Hunt-Shanks et al., 2009; Naqvi et al., 2005), on average, report being more depressed than their male counterparts. However, when it comes to heart failure, men report more distress and slower adjustment and recovery than women (Macabasco-O'Connell et al., 2010). Both women and blacks also are more likely to report being functionally limited by their illness compared to their white male counterparts. Future studies looking to replicate our efforts in understanding how individuals with CD live and age "with" it must, as such, strive to recruit samples that are more race and gender balanced.

References

Allen, M. (2017). *The Sage encyclopedia of communication research methods* (Vols. 1–4). Sage Publications, Inc. https://doi.org/10.4135/9781483381411

American Society for Gastrointestinal Endoscopy. (2018). https://www.asge.org/home/for-patients/conditions

Anderson, R. J., Freedland, K. E., Clouse, R. E., & Lustman, P. J. (2001). The prevalence of comorbid depression in adults with diabetes: A meta-analysis. *Diabetes Care, 24*(6), 1069–1078. https://doi.org/10.2337/diacare.23.7.934

Baider, L., Perez, T., & De-Nour, A. K. (1989). Gender and adjustment to chronic disease: A study of couples with colon cancer. *General Hospital Psychiatry, 11*(1), 1–8. https://doi.org/10.1016/0163-8343(89)90018-2

Barrett, A. E. (2003). Socioeconomic status and age identity: The role of dimensions of health in the subjective construction of age. *The Journals of Gerontology: Psychological Sciences and Social Sciences, 52B*, S101–S109. https://doi.org/10.1093/geronb/58.2.S101

Becker, G. (1997). *Disrupted lives: How people create meaning in a chaotic world.* University of California Press.

Benjamin Jr., A. J. (2020). Type A/B personalities. In B. J. Carducci, C. S. Nave, J. S. Mio, & R. E. Riggio (Eds.), *The Wiley encyclopedia of personality and individual differences: Clinical, applied, and cross-cultural research* (pp. 383–386). John Wiley & Sons. https://doi.org/10.1002/9781118970843.ch328

Berntsen, D., & Rubin, D. C. (2004). Cultural life scripts structure recall from autobiographical memory. *Memory & Cognition, 32*(3), 427–442. https://doi.org/10.3758/bf03195836

Bhattacherjee, A. (2012). *Social science research: Principles, methods, and practices.* Libre Texts. https://socialsci.libretexts.org/Bookshelves/Social_Work_and_Human_Services/Social_Science_Research_-_Principles_Methods_and_Practices_(Bhattacherjee)

Borawski, E. A., Kinney, J. M., & Kahana, E. (1996). The meaning of older adults' health appraisals: Congruence with health status and determinant of mortality. *Journal of Gerontological Social Work, 51B*, S157–S170.

Bowling, A., & Dieppe, P. (2005). What is successful ageing and who should define it? BMJ (Clinical research ed.), *331*(7531), 1548–1551. https://doi.org/10.1136/bmj.331.7531.1548

Bury, M. R. (2001). Illness narratives: Fact or fiction? *Sociology of Health and Illness, 23*, 253–285. https://doi.org/10.1111/1467-9566.00252

Butler, J. A., & Modaff, D. P. (2016). Motivations to disclose chronic illness in the workplace. *Qualitative Research Reports in Communication, 17*, 77–84. https://doi.org/10.1080/17459435.2016.1143387

Carstensen, L. L. (1992). Social and emotional patterns in adulthood: support for socio-emotional selectivity theory. *Psychology and Aging, 7*(3), 331–338.

Carstensen, L. L. (2006). The influence of a sense of time on human development. *Science, 312*, 1913–1915. https://doi.org/10.1126/science.1127488

Carstensen, L. L., Fung, H., & Charles, S.T. (2003). Socioemotional selectivity theory and emotion regulation in the second half of life. *Motivation and Emotion, 27*, 103–123.

Carstensen, L. L., Isaacowitz, D. M., & Charles, S. T. (1999). Taking time seriously: A theory of socioemotional selectivity. *American Psychologist, 54*(3), 165–181. https://doi.org/10.1037/0003-066X.54.3.165

Chapman, D. P., Perry, G. S., & Strine, T. W. (2005). Peer reviewed: The vital link between chronic disease and depressive disorders. *Preventing Chronic Disease, 2*(1), 1–10.

Charmaz, K. (1991). *Good days, bad days: The self in chronic illness and time.* Rutgers University Press.

Charmaz, K. (1999). Stories of suffering: Subjects' tales and research narratives. *Qualitative Health Research, 9*, 369–382.

Charmaz K. (2014). *Constructing grounded theory* (2nd ed.). Sage.

Cheng, S. T., Fuang, H., & Chan, A. (2007). Maintaining self-rated health through social comparison in old age. *The Journals of Gerontology (Series B, Psychological Sciences and Social Sciences), 62*(5), P277–P285. https://doi.org/10.1093/geronb/62.5.p277

Children's Health Defense (CHD). (2019). https://childrenshealthdefense.org/news/childrens-health/millennials-besieged-by-chronic-illness-from-age-27-its-all-downhill/

Clarke, L. H., & Korotchenko, A. (2011). Aging and the body: A review. *Canadian Journal on Aging = La Revue Canadienne du Vieillissement, 30*(3), 495–510. https://doi.org/10.1017/S0714980811000274

Cleaver, M., & Muller, T. E. (2002). I want to pretend I'm eleven years younger: Subjective age and seniors' motives for vacation travel. *Social Indicators Research, 60*(1/3), 227–41.

Cohen, N., & Arieli, T. (2011). Field research in conflict environments: Methodological challenges and snowball sampling. *Journal of Peace Resolution, 48*(4), 423–435.

Crohn's & Colitis Foundation of America. (n.d.). https://www.crohnscolitisfoundation.org/what-is-crohns-disease

Demakakos, P., Gjonca, E., & Nazroo, J. (2007). Age identity, age perceptions, and health: Evidence from the English longitudinal study of ageing. *Annals of the New York Academy of Sciences, 1114*, 279–287. https://doi.org/10.1196/annals.1396.021

Demmer, R. T., Gelb, S., Suglia, S. F., Keyes, K. M., Aiello, A. E., Colombo, P. C., Galea, S., Uddin, M., Koenen, K. C., & Kubzansky, L. D. (2015). Sex differences in the association between depression, anxiety, and type 2 diabetes mellitus. *Psychosomatic Medicine, 77*(4), 467–477. https://doi.org/10.1097/PSY.0000000000000169

Depp, C. A., & Jeste, D. V. (2006). Definitions and predictors of successful aging: A comprehensive review of larger quantitative studies. *The American Journal of Geriatric Psychiatry, 14*(1), 6–20. https://doi.org/10.1097/01.JGP.0000192501.03069.bc

DeVivo, M. J., & Chen, Y. (2011). Trends in new injuries, prevalent cases, and aging with spinal cord injury. *Archives of Physical Medicine and Rehabilitation, 92*, 332–338. https://doi.org/10.1016/j.apmr.2010.08.031

DeVivo, M. J., & Richards, J. S. (1996). Marriage rates among persons with spinal cord injury. *Rehabilitation Psychology, 41*, 321–339. https://doi.org/10.1037/h0092836

Erler, S. F., & Garstecki, D. C. (2002). Hearing loss- and hearing aid related stigma: Perceptions of women with age-normal hearing. *American Journal of Audiology, 11*, 83–91. https://doi.org/10.1044/1059-0889(2002/020)

Feigin, V., & GBD 2015 Risk Factors Collaborators. (2016). Global, regional, and national comparative risk assessment of behavioural, environmental and occupational, and metabolic risks or clusters of risks: A systematic analysis for the Global Burden of Disease Study 2015. *The Lancet, 388*(10053), 1659–1724.

Festinger, L. (1954). A theory of social comparison processes. *Human Relations, 7*(2), 117–140.

Feuerstein, J. D., & Cheifetz, A.S. (2017). Crohn disease: Epidemiology, diagnosis, and management. *Mayo Clinic Proceedings, 92*(7), 1088–1103. https://doi.org/10.1016/j.mayocp.2017.04.010

Folkman, S., Lazarus, R. S., Pimley, S., & Novacek, J. (1987). Age differences in stress and coping processes. *Psychology and Aging*, 2, 171–184.

Foucault, M. (1980). *Power/knowledge: Selected interviews and other writings, 1972–1977*. Vintage.

Fredrickson, B. L., & Carstensen, L. L. (1990). Choosing social partners: How old age and anticipated endings make people more selective. *Psychology and Aging, 5*(3), 335–337. https://doi.org/10.1037/0882-7974.5.3.335

Frieswijk, N., Buunk, B. P., Steverink, N., & Slaets, J. P. (2004). The interpretation of social comparison and its relation to life satisfaction among elderly people: Does frailty make a difference?. *The Journals of Gerontology (Series B, Psychological Sciences and Social Sciences), 59*(5), P250–P257. https://doi.org/10.1093/geronb/59.5.p250

Fung, H. H., Carstensen, L. L., & Lutz, A. M. (1999). Influence of time on social preferences: Implications for life-span development. *Psychology and Aging, 14*(4), 595–604.

Gecas, V. (1989). The social-psychology of self-efficacy. *Annual Review of Sociology, 15*, 291–316.

Geronimus A. T. (1992). The weathering hypothesis and the health of African-American women and infants: Evidence and speculations. *Ethnicity & disease, 2*(3), 207–221.

Glaser, B. G., Strauss, A. L., & Strutzel, E. (1968). The discovery of grounded theory; Strategies for qualitative research. *Nursing Research, 17*(4), 364.

Heidrich, S. M., & Ryff, C. D. (1993a). Physical and mental health in later life: The self-system as mediator. *Psychology and Aging, 8*, 327–338. https://doi.org/10.1037/0882-7974.8.3.327

Heidrich, S. M., & Ryff, C. D. (1993b). The role of social comparisons processes in the psychological adaptation of elderly adults. *Journal of Gerontology, 48*, 127–136. https://doi.org/10.1093/geronj/48.3.P127

Helgeson, V. S. (2017). Young adults with type 1 diabetes: Romantic relationships and implications for well-being. *Diabetes Spectrum, 30*(2), 108–116. https://doi.org/10.2337/ds16-0020

Hubley, A. M., & Russell, L. B. (2009). Prediction of subjective age, desired age, and age satisfaction in older adults: Do some health dimensions contribute more than others? *International Journal of Behavioral Development, 33*(1), 12–21. https://doi.org/10.1177/0165025408099486

Hunt-Shanks, T., Blanchard, C., & Reid, R. D. (2009). Gender differences in cardiac patients: A longitudinal investigation of exercise, autonomic anxiety, negative affect and depression. *Psychology, Health & Medicine, 14*(3), 375–385. https://doi.org/10.1080/13548500902866939

Huygens, M. W., Vermeulen, J., Swinkels, I. C., Friele, R. D., van Schayck, O. C., & de Witte, L. P. (2016). Expectations and needs of patients with a chronic disease toward self-management and eHealth for self-management purposes. *BMC Health Services Research, 16*, 232. https://doi.org/10.1186/s12913-016-1484-5

Ishige, T. (2019). Growth failure in pediatric onset inflammatory bowel disease: Mechanisms, epidemiology, and management. *Translational Pediatrics, 8*(1), 16–22. https://doi.org/10.21037/tp.2018.12.04

Katz, S., & Calasanti, T. (2015). Critical perspectives on successful aging: Does it "appeal more than it illuminates"? *The Gerontologist, 55*(1), 26–33. https://doi.org/10.1093/geront/gnu027

Keller, R. M., & Galgay, C. E. (2010). Microaggressive experiences of people with disabilities. In D. W. Sue (Ed.), *Microaggressions and marginality: Manifestation, dynamics, and impact* (pp. 241–268). Wiley & Sons.

Kotter-Grühn, D., Kleinspehn-Ammerlahn, A., Gerstorf, D., & Smith, J. (2009). Self-perceptions of aging predict mortality and change with approaching death: 16-year longitudinal results from the Berlin Aging Study. *Psychology and Aging, 24*, 654–667. https://doi.org/10.1037/a0016510

Kwak, S., Kim, H., Chey, J., & Youm, Y. (2018). Feeling how old I am: Subjective age is associated with estimated brain age. *Frontiers in Aging Neuroscience, 10*, 1–10. https://doi.org/10.3389/fnagi.2018.00168

LaDonna, K. A., Ghavanini, A. A., & Venance, S. L. (2015). Truths and misinformation: A qualitative exploration of myotonic dystrophy. *The Canadian Journal of Neurological Sciences, 42*(3), 187–194. https://doi.org/10.1017/cjn.2015.26

Leray, E., Moreau, T., Fromont, A., & Edan, G. (2016). Epidemiology of multiple sclerosis. *Revue Neurologique, 172*, 3–13. https://doi.org/10.1016/j.neurol.2015.10.006

Li, C., Ford, E. S., Strine, T. W., & Mokdad, A. H. (2008). Prevalence of depression among US adults with diabetes: Findings from the 2006 behavioral risk factor surveillance system. *Diabetes Care, 31*(1), 105–107. https://doi.org/10.2337/dc07-1154

Linden, W., Vodermaier, A., Mackenzie, R., & Greig, D. (2012). Anxiety and depression after cancer diagnosis: Prevalence rates by cancer type, gender, and age. *Journal of Affective Disorders, 141*(2–3), 343–351. https://doi.org/10.1016/j.jad.2012.03.025

Liu Jr., J. L., & Richardson, P. K. (2012). Successful aging in older adults with disability. *OTJR: Occupation, Participation and Health, 32*(4), 126–134. https://doi.org/10.3928/15394492-20120203-02

Marks, R. (2018). Successful aging and chronic osteoarthritis. *Medicines (Basel, Switzerland), 5*(3), 105. https://doi.org/10.3390/medicines5030105

Marrie, R. A., Yu, N., Blanchard, J., Leung, S., & Elliott, L. (2010). The rising prevalence and changing age distribution of multiple sclerosis in Manitoba. *Neurology, 74*, 465–471. https://doi.org/10.1212/WNL.0b013e3181cf6ec0

Martinson, M., & Berridge, C. (2015). Successful aging and its discontents: A systematic review of the social gerontology literature. *The Gerontologist, 55*(1), 58–69. https://doi.org/10.1093/geront/gnu037

Macabasco-O'Connell, A., Crawford, M. H., Stotts, N., Stewart, A., & Froelicher, E. S. (2010). Gender and racial differences in psychosocial factors of low-income patients with heart failure. *Heart & Lung, 39*(1), 2–11. https://doi.org/10.1016/j.hrtlng.2009.05.001

McGonagle, A. K., & Barnes-Farrell, J. (2014). Chronic illness in the workplace: Stigma, identity threat, and strain. *Stress and Health, 30*, 310–321. https://doi.org/10.1002/smi.2518

Menec, V. H., & Perry, R. P. (1995). Reactions to stigmas: The effect of targets' age and controllability of stigmas. *Journal of Aging and Health*, 7, 365–383.

Miserandino, C. (2003). *The spoon theory*. www.butyoudontlooksick.com/the_spoon_theory

Molton, I., & Yorkston, K. (2017). Growing older with physical disability: A special application of the successful aging paradigm. *Journals of Gerontology: Social Sciences*. https://doi.org10.1093/geronb/gbw122

Naqvi, T. Z., Naqvi, S. S., & Merz, C. N. (2005). Gender differences in the link between depression and cardiovascular disease. *Psychosomatic Medicine, 67*(Suppl. 1), S15–S18. https://doi.org/10.1097/01.psy.0000164013.55453.05

NCHS. (n.d.). *Technical notes for summary health statistics tables: National health interview survey*. CDC. https://www.cdc.gov/nchs/nhis/SHS/tables.htm

Neugarten, B. L. (1968). Adult personality: Toward a psychology of the life cycle. In B. L. Neugarten (Ed.), *Middle age and aging: A reader in social psychology* (pp. 137–147). University of Chicago Press.

Neugarten B. L., Moore J. W., & Lowe J. C. (1965). Age norms, age constraints, and adult socialization. *American Journal of Sociology, 70*, 710–717.

Noonan, V. K., Fingas, M., Farry, A., Baxter, D., Singh, A., Fehlings, M. G., & Dvorak, M. F. (2012). Incidence and prevalence of spinal cord injury in Canada: A national perspective. *Neuroepidemiology*, *38*, 219–226. https://doi.org/10.1159/000336014

Nowakowski, A. C. (2016). Hope is a four-letter word: Riding the emotional rollercoaster of illness management. *Sociology of Health & Illness*, *38*(6), 899–915. https://doi.org/10.1111/1467-9566.12403

Öberg, P., & Tornstam, L. (2001). Youthfulness and fitness—Identity ideals for all ages? *Journal of Aging & Identity*, *6*(1), 15–29.

Palinkas, L. A., Horwitz, S. M., Green, C. A., Wisdom, J. P., Duan, N., & Hoagwood, K. (2015). Purposeful sampling for qualitative data collection and analysis in mixed method implementation research. *Administration and Policy in Mental Health*, *42*(5), 533–544. https://doi.org/10.1007/s10488-013-0528-y

Park, S. C., & Jeen, Y. T. (2019). Genetic studies of inflammatory bowel disease-focusing on Asian patients. *Cells*, *8*(5), 404. https://doi.org/10.3390/cells8050404

Pecchioni, L. L. (2012). Interruptions to cultural life scripts: Cancer diagnoses, contextual age, and life narratives. *Research on Aging*, *34*(6), 758–780. https://doi.org/10.1177/0164027512449748

Pebdani, R. N., Johnson, K. L., Amtmann, D., Bamer, A. M., & Wundes, A. (2015). Experiences and perspectives of pregnancy in women with multiple sclerosis. *Sexuality and Disability*, *33*(1), 47–52.

Phelan, E. A., & Larson, E. B. (2002). "Successful aging"—Where next? *Journal of the American Geriatric Society*, *50*, 1306–1308. https://doi.org/10.1046/j.1532-5415.2002.50324.x

Piazza, J. R., Charles, S. T., & Almeida, D. M. (2007). Living with chronic health conditions: Age differences in affective well-being. *The Journals of Gerontology* (*Series B, Psychological Sciences and Social Sciences*), *62*(6), 313–321. https://doi.org/10.1093/geronb/62.6.p313

QSR International Pty Ltd. Version 11. (2015). NVivo qualitative data analysis software. https://lumivero.com/products/nvivo/

Reeuwijk, K. G., van Klaveren, D., van Rijn, R. M., Burdorf, A., & Robroek, S. J. (2017). The influence of poor health on competing exit routes from paid employment among older workers in 11 European countries. *Scandinavian Journal of Work, Environment & Health*, *43*(1), 24–33. https://doi.org/10.5271/sjweh.3601

Rejeski, W. J., Miller, M. E., Foy, C. G., Messier, S. P., & Rapp, S. (2001). Self-efficacy and the progression of functional limitations and self-reported disability in older adults with knee pain. *The Journals of Gerontology* (*Series B: Psychological Sciences and Social Sciences*), *56*, 261–265. https://doi.org/10.1093/geronb/56.5.S261

Rosen, M. J., Dhawan, A., & Saeed, S. A. (2015). Inflammatory bowel disease in children and adolescents. *JAMA Pediatrics*, *169*(11), 1053–1060. https://doi.org/10.1001/jamapediatrics.2015.1982

Saadeh, M., Welmer, A. K., Dekhtyar, S., Fratiglioni, L., & Calderón Larrañaga, A. (2020). The role of psychological and social well-being on physical function trajectories in older adults. *The Journals of Gerontology (Series A, Biological Sciences and Medical Sciences)*, *75*(8), 1579–1585. https://doi.org/10.1093/gerona/glaa114

Sanders, C., Donovan, J., & Dieppe, P. (2002). The significance and consequences of having painful and disabled joints in older age: Co-existing accounts of normal and disrupted biographies, *Sociology of Health and Illness*, *24*, 227–253. https://doi.org/10.1111/1467-9566.00292

Scalfari, A., Knappertz, V., Cutter, G., Goodin, D. S., Ashton, R., & Ebers, G. C. (2013). Mortality in patients with multiple sclerosis. *Neurology*, *81*(2), 184–192. https://doi.org/10.1212/WNL.0b013e31829a3388

Schofield, D. J., Callander, E. J., Shrestha, R. N., Passey, M. E., Percival, R., & Kelly, S. J. (2012). Association between co-morbidities and labour force participation amongst persons with back problems. *Pain*, *153*(10), 2068–2072. https://doi.org/10.1016/j.pain.2012.06.020

Schuring, M., Robroek, S. J., Otten, F. W., Arts, C. H., & Burdorf, A. (2013). The effect of ill health and socioeconomic status on labor force exit and re-employment: A prospective study with ten years follow-up in the Netherlands. *Scandinavian Journal of Work, Environment and Health*, *39*(2), 134–143. https://doi.org/10.5271/sjweh.3321

Smith, G. (2008). *Does gender influence online survey participation? A record-linkage analysis of university faculty online survey response behavior.* ERIC Document Reproduction Service No. ED 501717.

Smith, K. J., Deschênes, S. S., & Schmitz, N. (2018). Investigating the longitudinal association between diabetes and anxiety: A systematic review and meta-analysis. *Diabetic Medicine: A Journal of the British Diabetic Association*, *35*(6), 677–693. https://doi.org/10.1111/dme.13606

Staudinger, U. M. (2015). Images of aging: Outside and inside perspectives. *Annual Review of Gerontology and Geriatrics*, *35*, 187–209. https://doi.org/10.1891/0198-8794.35.29

Stephan, Y., Caudroit J., & Chalabaev A. (2011). Subjective health and memory self-efficacy as mediators in the relation between subjective age and life satisfaction among older adults. *Aging & Mental Health*, *15*, 428–436. https://doi.org/10.1080/13607863.2010.536138

Stephan, Y., Chalabaev, A., Kotter-Grühn, D., & Jaconelli, A. (2013). "Feeling younger, being stronger": An experimental study of subjective age and physical functioning among older adults. *Journals of Gerontology (Series B: Psychological Sciences and Social Sciences)*, *68*, 1–7. https://doi.org/10.1093/geronb/gbs037

Stephan, Y., Sutin, A. R., Bayard, S., & Terracciano, A. (2017). Subjective age and sleep in middle-aged and older adults. *Psychology & Health*, *32*(9), 1140–1151. https://doi.org/10.1080/08870446.2017.1324971

Stephan, Y., Sutin, A. R., Luchetti, M., & Terracciano, A. (2017). Feeling older and the development of cognitive impairment and dementia. *Journals of Gerontology (Series B: Psychological Sciences and Social Sciences)*, *72*(6), 966–973. https://doi.org/10.1093/geronb/gbw085

Stephan, Y., Sutin, A. R., & Terracciano, A. (2016). Feeling older and risk of hospitalization: Evidence from three longitudinal cohorts. *Health Psychology*, *35*(6), 634. https://doi.org/10.1037/hea0000335

Stephan, Y., Sutin, A. R., & Terracciano, A. (2018). Subjective age and mortality in three longitudinal samples. *Psychosomatic Medicine*, *80*(7), 659–664. https://doi.org/10.1097/PSY.0000000000000613

Strauss, D. J., Devivo, M. J., Paculdo, D. R., & Shavelle, R. M. (2006). Trends in life expectancy after spinal cord injury. *Archives of Physical Medicine and Rehabilitation*, *87*, 1079–1085. https://doi.org/10.1016/j.apmr.2006.04.022

Strauss, D., Shavelle, R., Reynolds, R., Rosenbloom, L., & Day, S. (2007). Survival in cerebral palsy in the last 20 years: Signs of improvement? *Developmental Medicine & Child Neurology*, *49*, 86–92. https://doi.org/10.1111/j.1469-8749.2007.00086.x

Strawbridge, W. J., Wallhagen, M. I., & Cohen, R. D. (2002). Successful aging and well-being: Self-rated compared with Rowe and Kahn. *The Gerontologist*, *42*(6), 727–733. https://doi.org/10.1093/geront/42.6.727

Sullivan-Singh, S. J., Stanton, A. L., & Low, C. A. (2015). Living with limited time: Socioemotional selectivity theory in the context of health adversity. *Journal of Personality and Social Psychology*, *108*(6), 900–916. https://doi.org/10.1037/a0039047

Tay, J., Goss, A. M., Locher, J. L., Ard, J. D., & Gower, B. A. (2019). Physical function and strength in relation to inflammation in older adults with obesity and increased cardiometabolic risk. *The Journal of Nutrition, Health and Aging*, *23*(10), 949–957. https://doi.org/10.1007/s12603-019-1260-4

Torres, J., Mehandru, S., Colombel J. F., & Peyrin-Biroulet, L. (2017). Crohn's disease. *Lancet*, *389*, 1741–1755. https://doi.org/10.1016/S0140-6736(16)31711-1

Transamerica Health Studies Center. (2016). https://www.transamericacenterforhealthstudies.org/

Turner, B. (1984). *The body and society: Explorations in social theory*. Basil Blackwell.

Turner, J., & Kelly, B. (2000). Emotional dimensions of chronic disease. *The Western Journal of Medicine*, *172*(2), 124–128. https://doi.org/10.1136/ewjm.172.2.124

Ubel, P. A., Jankovic, A., Smith, D., Langa, K. M., & Fagerlin, A. (2005). What is perfect health to an 85-year-old? Evidence for scale recalibration in subjective health ratings. *Medical Care*, *43*(10), 1054–1057. https://doi.org/10.1097/01.mlr.0000178193.38413.70

Van Rijn, R. M., Robroek, S. J., Brouwer, S., & Burdorf, A. (2014). Influence of poor health on exit from paid employment: A systematic review. *Occupational and Environmental Medicine*, *71*(4), 295–301.

Verbrugge, L. M., & Yang, L. (2002) Aging with disability and disability with aging. *Journal of Disability Policy Studies, 12*(40), 253–267. https://doi.org/10.1177/104420730201200405

West, M. D., Dye, A. N., & McMahon, B. T. (2006). Epilepsy and workplace discrimination: population characteristics and trends. *Epilepsy & Behavior: E&B, 9*(1), 101–105. https://doi.org/10.1016/j.yebeh.2006.03.011

Wilkinson, H. R., & Nair, R. D. (2013). The psychological impact of the unpredictability of multiple sclerosis: A qualitative literature meta-synthesis. *British Journal of Neuroscience Nursing, 9*(4), 172–178. https://doi.org/10.12968/bjnn.2013.9.4.172

Williamson, G. M., Schulz, R. (1995). Symptoms of depression in elderly persons: Beyond the effects of physical illness and disability. In B. J. Vellas, J. L. Albarede, & P. J. Potter (Eds.), *Mood and cognitive disorders. Facts and research in gerontology* (pp. 9–19). Springer.

Wolff, J. L., Starfield, B., & Anderson, G. (2002). Prevalence, expenditures, and complications of multiple chronic conditions in the elderly. *Journal of the American Medical Association, 162*, 2269–2276. https://doi.org/10.1001/archinte.162.20.2269

Wright, B., & Schwager, P. H. (2008). Onlin survey research: Can response factors be improved? *Journal of Internet Commerce, 7*(2), 253–269.

CHAPTER 2

A Case Study of BIPOC Spouses with Rare and Genetic Diseases

Michele Wise Wright and Terry Gene Wright

The topic of "Aging Invisibly" is an interesting one, because it so often signifies how we can age with beauty, grace, and eloquence. It also eludes to not being able to see or at least minimize the physical (visible) attributes quite often associated with aging such as wrinkles and scars. But if people could actually see our invisible scars, cuts, and bruises, then how much more powerfully would our real story, challenges, pains, and triumphs be revealed.

So, is the case with spouses, Michele and Terry Wright, married November 4, 2000. Little did they know upon meeting on November 1, 1999, that not only would they connect in love but in aging invisibly. Interestingly enough, they would also both earn their purple ribbons, in a 1:2 ratio for Systemic Lupus Erythematosus (Lupus) and Cystic Fibrosis (CF), respectfully. The 1:2 ratio is very unique to Michele and Terry.

Michele was born in the month of April (4) and Terry was born in the month of August (8), a 1:2 ratio. Michele was born on the 8th day of April (8) and Terry was born on the 16th day of August (16), another 1:2 ratio. And when it came to being diagnosed with rare and genetic diseases, Michele was diagnosed with Lupus at the age of 27 and Terry was diagnosed with CF at the age of 54, yet another interesting 1:2 ratio that would not only connect them in love, but in sickness and in health.

As noted earlier, the purple ribbon is ironically the symbol for both Lupus and CF, not to mention that the month of May is the official awareness month for both diseases. This is important to Michele and Terry as it allows them to not only own their conditions but make them visible as an inspiration and symbol of hope to others dealing with a rare and genetic disease, so that they can proudly display their ribbons as well. Thus, these ribbons are not only a representation of survival but strength and courage. As noted under pulse uniform:[1]

> In the healthcare sector, the use of colored ribbons helps in creating public awareness to disability, medical conditions, health and other issues. An awareness ribbon is simply a short piece of colored ribbon that is

 | DOI:10.1163/9789004708136_003

folded in a loop. These ribbons are adorned by people from all over the globe such as United States, United Kingdom, Canada, Australia, etc. as a support for the issue or cause.

While you may have seen an awareness ribbon, you may not be aware of how many they are, the different colors and patterns they represent. Over the passage of time, new awareness ribbons are being created each day in support of hundreds of causes.

You will encounter a variety of awareness ribbons in your day-to-day encounters, where each means something different from the other. For instance, green is in support for an environmental cause, red is for coronary diseases, blue is for bullying awareness, etc. Regardless of the color of the ribbon, the idea remains the same…

The purpose behind these ribbons is to eradicate an illness and support the struggle of a loved on. Thereby, all efforts despite how big or small, bring us a step closer to the innate goal. In the healthcare industry, it is important to have a supportive network of allies that understand your struggle and vision.

The history of awareness ribbons is not clear, but they take roots from the practices followed in medieval times when ladies gave knights their token of affection and love. A few people believe that ribbons first gained popularity in the United States during the Civil War. Women wore yellow ribbons to express gratitude for loved ones on the battlefield.

While there is little evidence regarding the Civil War theory, it was the first time that yellow ribbons were used in the United States. The first time in November 1979, Penney Laingen tied a yellow ribbon on a tree outside her house in support of Ambassador Bruce Laingen, her husband who had been taken hostage by Iranian revolutionaries when the American embassy was seized in Tehran. Her inspiration for this gesture was the old song, "Tie a Yellow Ribbon Round the Ole Oak Tree."

Laingen and other hostages were then released in January 1981, but the awareness ribbons were meant to stay. The yellow ribbons are worn as a support for the soldiers at war in the United States. However, it may have different meanings in other parts of the world.

Of course, you can wear a ribbon on its own, but there are also others ways to show your support for a cause. For example, breast cancer is an extremely popular cause that is supported with pink ribbons.

Since many awareness campaigns share the same color or have various alternate colors, it is important to learn what cause you are actually supporting.

This brings us back to the purple ribbons. As @pulseuniform (2018) continues:

> Purple typically represents pancreatic cancer and epilepsy. It is also a symbol for Alzheimer's disease, *lupus*, animal abuse, Crohn's disease, *cystic fibrosis*, fibromyalgia, sarcoidosis awareness, thyroid cancer, ADD (Attention Deficit Disorder), and religious tolerance.
>
> – *Lavender*: Caregiver Appreciation, Cancer (unspecified), Epilepsy, Gynecological Cancer, Foster Care, Infantile Spasms, Hypokalemic Periodic Paralysis, Rett Syndrome
> – *Orchid*: Testicular Cancer
> – *Purple*: ADHD, Animal Abuse, Crohn's Disease, ADD, Arnold Chiari Malformation, Alzheimer's, Anti-Violence, Fibromyalgia in Men, GI Cancer (Intestinal), Chronic Pain, Colitis, Cystic Fibrosis, Epilepsy, Fibromyalgia, Harmony, Homelessness, Leiomyosarcoma, Lupus, Mucolipidosis, Neuropathy Awareness, Macular Degeneration, Migraines (1st choice: alternate burgundy), Domestic Violence, No Unattended Kids in Cars, Pancreatic Cancer, Pancreatitis (Chronic), Thyroid Cancer, Religious Tolerance, Mesh Survivor, Sarcoidosis, Sjogren's Syndrome, Thymoma Cancer, Rett Syndrome, Victims of 9/11
> – *Violet Ribbon*: Hodgkin's Disease, Testicular Cancer.

Transitioning back to Michele and Terry, it is important to understand the significance of their specific purple ribbons and disease states, Lupus and Cystic Fibrosis.

1 Lupus

The Lupus Foundation of America,[2] the largest force in the fight to cure lupus, defines lupus as a chronic (long-term) disease that can cause inflammation

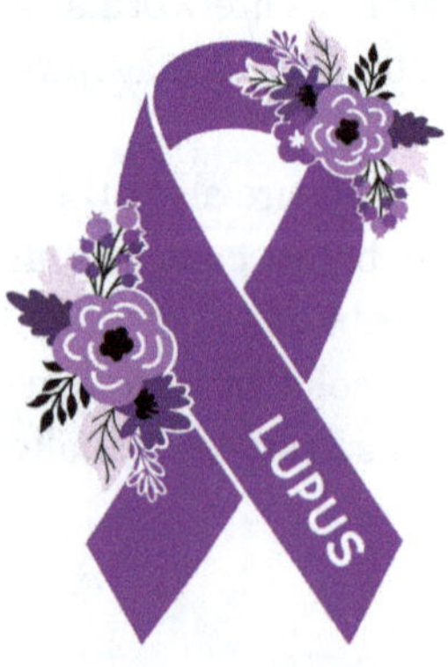

FIGURE 2.1
Purple lupus ribbon (@SpoonieSisterShop)[3]

and pain in any part of your body. It's an autoimmune disease, which means that your immune system—the body system that usually fights infections—attacks healthy tissue instead. Lupus most commonly affects your: Skin, Joints, and Internal organs, like your kidneys and heart. Because lupus affects many parts of the body, it can cause a lot of different symptoms. The organization expounds,

> When people talk about lupus, they're usually talking about *systemic lupus*. But there are four kinds of lupus: Systemic lupus erythematosus (SLE), the most common form of lupus; Cutaneous lupus, a form of lupus that is limited to the skin; Drug-induced lupus, a lupus-like disease caused by certain prescription drugs; and Neonatal lupus, a rare condition that affects infants of women who have lupus.

2 Cystic Fibrosis

According to the Cystic Fibrosis Foundation (CFF),[4] the world's leader in the search for a cure, funding promising research and working to provide access to quality, specialized care and treatments for people with cystic fibrosis (CF), CF is a genetic disorder that affects the lungs, pancreas, and other organs, and how to treat and live with this chronic disease. CFF explains,

> In people with CF, mutations in the cystic fibrosis transmembrane conductance regulator (CFTR) gene cause the CFTR protein to become dysfunctional. When the protein is not working correctly, it's unable to help move chloride—a component of salt—to the cell surface. Without the chloride to attract water to the cell surface, the mucus in various organs becomes thick and sticky.

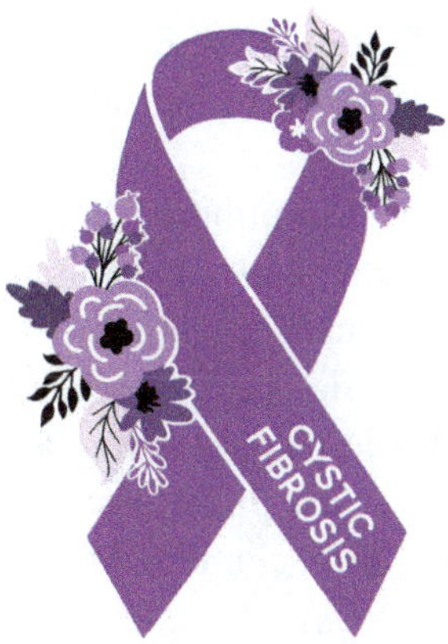

FIGURE 2.2
Purple cystic fibrosis ribbon (@SpoonieSisterShop)[5]

And now Michele and Terry wear purple not only for each other but to make an individual, collective, and synergistic difference in each of these distinguished communities. However, although their ribbons are similar in color, as members of the community of Black, Indigenous and people of color (BIPOC), their individualized journeys with each of diseases have been distinctively different and remarkable. Following is a case study of Michele and Terry's journey, as BIPOC spouses, with rare (lupus) and genetic (cystic fibrosis) diseases.

3 Michele Wright, Ph.D., African American (BIPOC) Woman with Rare Disease Systemic Lupus Erythematosus (SLE)

Michele Wright was born Michele Rhonda Wise on April 8, 1966 in Tuskegee, Alabama to parents Frankie and Garland Wise. She was born at the John A. Andrew Memorial Hospital, a former teaching hospital that was located directly on the campus of Tuskegee Institute/Tuskegee University during its years of operation from 1892–1987. This is also the same hospital that the infamous Tuskegee Study of Untreated Syphilis in the Negro Male took place. As the Centers for Disease Control and Prevention (CDC) states:[6]

> In 1932, the USPHS, working with the Tuskegee Institute, began a study to record the natural history of syphilis. It was originally called the "Tuskegee Study of Untreated Syphilis in the Negro Male" (now referred to as the "USPHS Syphilis Study at Tuskegee"). The study initially involved 600 Black men—399 with syphilis, 201 who did not have the disease. Participants' informed consent was not collected. Researchers told the men they were being treated for "bad blood," a local term used to describe several ailments, including syphilis, anemia, and fatigue. In exchange for taking part in the study, the men received free medical exams, free meals, and burial insurance.
>
> By 1943, penicillin was the treatment of choice for syphilis and becoming widely available, but the participants in the study were not offered treatment.
>
> In 1972, an Associated Press story about the study was published. As a result, the Assistant Secretary for Health and Scientific Affairs appointed an Ad Hoc Advisory Panel to review the study. The advisory panel concluded that the study was "ethically unjustified;" that is, the "results [were] disproportionately meager compared with known risks to human subjects involved." In October 1972, the panel advised stopping the study. A month later, the Assistant Secretary for Health and Scientific Affairs

> announced the end of the study. In March 1973, the panel also advised the Secretary of the Department of Health, Education, and Welfare (HEW) (now known as the Department of Health and Human Services) to instruct the USPHS to provide all necessary medical care for the survivors of the study. The Tuskegee Health Benefit Program (THBP) was established to provide these services.
>
> In 1975, participants' wives, widows and children were added to the program. In 1995, the program was expanded to include health, as well as medical, benefits. The last study participant died in January 2004. The last widow receiving THBP benefits died in January 2009.
>
> Participants' children (10 at present) continue to receive medical and health benefits.
>
> Later in 1973, a class-action lawsuit was filed on behalf of the study participants and their families, resulting in a $10 million, out-of-court settlement in 1974.
>
> On May 16, 1997, President Bill Clinton issued a formal apology for the study.

But the informally known "Tuskegee Syphilis Study" is considered among a plethora of historical events/people that Tuskegee has become known for including the Tuskegee Airmen, Booker T. Washington, George Washington Carver, Rosa Parks, Lionel Richie, the Commodores, Tom Joyner, and of course, Michele (Wise) Wright who historical roadmap is uniquely documented and celebrated in its own right.

Michele is the second oldest of five siblings. Growing up, she dealt with a severe speech impediment that often made it difficult for her to be heard or understood. After taking speech therapy for many years, she declined to continue once high school approached. In high school, she had a deep love for dance and even desire to be a solid gold dancer. But she also had a late discovery of love for Mathematics. When it was time to determine her path in life, Michele thought dance and her dad thought engineering. In the end engineering prevailed and she exceeded greatly.

She received a cooperative education scholarship that allowed her to attend Tuskegee University for a semester and then work in the field of engineering (with a reputable organization) another semester. In 1990, Michele graduated from Tuskegee University as electrical engineering student of the year and decided to continue her education in engineering. She applied and subsequently received the esteemed National GEM Consortium's graduate engineering and science fellowship program (GEM). Thus, in 1990, she entered the University of Tennessee Space Institute (UTSI) as the first GEM fellow in the

UTSI's history as a graduate student in engineering management/industrial engineering.

As a GEM Fellow, Michele would attend school during the regular school year and intern with a reputable engineering company during the summer months. In May 1992, she made history as the first full-time African American student to earn a master's degree in engineering management from the UTSI. It appeared Engineering was her destiny, especially the job offers that followed including several from Fortune 100 companies. Thus, nothing appeared to stand in the way of the top-notch engineering career that Michele so diligently pursue. That was until she stepped into her first job with a Fortune 50 company and began not only her career as an engineer but, soon afterwards, her unforeseen journey with lupus.

Michele was optimistic about her new title as Distribution Center Project Engineer. However, barely a year within her post, she began experiencing an array of strange events including extreme tiredness and fatigue, severe joint pain and stiffness, low-grade fever, skins lesions and rashes, dry eyes and mouth, shortness of breath, chest pain and anxiety, fingers and toes that would turn blue upon cold exposure, and headaches and confusion.

As a project engineer who had to cover a lot of ground physically and mentally, these strange and unexplained events were a cause for great concerned. Michele worked hard for years to get to her level of career and didn't want any unforeseen event to impact her quality of work, performance, and success. She even wondered if the stress of her job was causing all of these occurrences to be in her mind. But being an engineer, Michele knew something wasn't technically adding up and that all these signs and symptoms could not be simply a fragment of her imagination.

To make matters worse, Michele began losing a lot of weight and found it difficult to keep an appetite. She also had occasional blood and mucus in her stools and her fingers appeared to become disformed. So, after finding it more and more difficult to walk, breath, and move, she finally sought medical help and answers. After not finding many answers with a first physician, she was fortunate the second go around. Following her examination (February 4, 1994), the internist informed Michele that he believed she had lupus.

Lupus was unfortunately a term she was accustomed to because she previously lost a high school classmate and high school teacher from lupus. She also recalled the devastating lesions that resembled third degree burns on both of these individual faces. She thought to herself, "I can't have lupus. This would be a death sentence." The doctor scheduled her to return on February 14, 1994 to receive the final results. Michele smirked and left this physician's office to run downstairs to the closest payphone booth to call her mother collect. She accepted the phone call but not the news. Her mom told her that the doctor was wrong and that it is no way she could have lupus. They were both for the moment in complete denial.

This all changed on Valentine's Day 1994 when the doctor stepped back into the examination room and immediately told Michele that his suspicions were correct that she indeed had systemic lupus erythematosus, an autoimmune and inflammatory disease that exists when the immune system attacks its own tissues, organs, etc. She was speechless and the trip to the phone booth seemed forever away. She managed nonetheless and broke the upsetting news (via a collect call) to her mother as they both sat in silence.

Finally, her mother assured her that everything was going to be alright and to stay encouraged. This would be all the more difficult to do as both time and lupus progressed. Within several months, Michele went from bad to worse. She found it near impossible to stand and walk from the unbearable pain and weakness in her joints and muscles. She also continued to lose weight and the blood and mucus in her bowels were becoming more evident. Her skin coloring also started to become ashy.

After being referred to a gastroenterologist and hospitalized, it was determined that she had colon vasculitis, a vasculitis and/or ischemia of the small intestine or colon. In an attempt to save her life, her GI put her on high dose prednisone, which belongs to a class of drugs known as corticosteroids (a type of anti-inflammatory drug commonly referred to as steroids) and came with its own bag of issues. According to Everyday Health,[7]

> But prednisone comes with a range of unwelcome side effects, one of which is weight gain.
>
> According to a study published in January 2020 in the journal *Lung*, participants taking prednisone reported increased appetite resulting in weight gain. And a review published n February 2021 in the journal *Obesity* noted that long-term prednisone use affected body weight, appetite, and body composition.
>
> Weight gain from prednisone often appears as fat deposits on various parts of your body, such as at the base or back of your neck, around your abdomen, or as what's called "moon face," when changes in where fat lies make your face appear rounder and wider.

Michele inevitably gained about 50 pounds and her extreme round (moon) face made her not only unrecognizable but ashamed to be seen in public. She vividly remembers being in a store where one of her co-workers came by and didn't recognize her. The woman asked her if they knew each other and

Michele began to sobbed uncontrollably. At that moment, which was not only dealing with the physical and transformational side effects of her condition and treatment, but the sociological and psychological affects with struggling with her own sense of self identity changing. Michele no longer saw herself as a confident woman of beauty to be admire but an insecure woman of shame who wanted to hide from the world. But Michele had bigger concerns than pure vanity. Rather, she was in a fight for her very life.

Michele was eventually referred to a rheumatologist who was shocked by the high daily dose of the powerful anti-inflammatory corticosteroids she was taking. He said, "We got to get you off this medicine little by little and put you on Imuran and Plaquenil." Although relieved, she was still discouraged about her quality of life—or having much of a life at all. Although Michele knew she was fighting for her life, she also knew she could not continue this battle alone. This is when her father made arrangements for her mother to travel from Tuskegee to help nurse Michele back to health. This process involved preparing and cooking Michele some of her favorite childhood meals (i.e., chicken, dressing, greens, cornbread, rice pudding, banana pudding, and pound cake) as well as getting her up to walk everyday (even if only for a few feet at first). It worked. Upon her mother arriving, Michele began eating again and trying to get some level of physical activity including walking, a lifelong favorite of hers, so that she could return back to work as soon as possible. Walking was beneficial both physically and mentally to her because growing up it was something she always did as bonding time with her mother and father. Walking also allowed her to get out of the house and enjoy the beautiful sights of nature and atmosphere of simply being outside. It was her path towards walking back to normalcy.

In reality, Michele's healing process was slow and painful and the devastating results of deep and enduring injustices in accessibility for people with disabling chronic conditions. Consequently, these interlocking systems of power and inequality impacted not only her health but her demanding career as an engineer. She had many changes she desired to make that were an integral part of her journey back to finding self. This included finding the energy to want to get out of bed every day to perform the daily activities of life (i.e., bathing, dressing, eating). It also involved cultivating a positive attitude and gratefulness to simply see another day. Furthermore, it required learning to integrate herself back into the public in lieu of hiding at every opportunity possibly. After an extensive healing process, she decided to transition in career and location. She ultimately relocated to Arkansas to start a new position in sales.

Following this change of direction, Michele felt heartened to see how engineering and her critical thinking skills remained an integral part of her various tasks, duties, and responsibilities. This move proved to be one of the best decisions of her career and life. Michele soared to the top and received the prestigious Eagle award for her first sales position in food sales.

Michele's success continued during her transition to the field of pharmaceutical & biotechnology sales, where she excelled to the top of sales achievement and excellence (winning both top International/National awards) with top ranked corporations including Pfizer Pharmaceuticals, Novartis Pharmaceuticals, and Genentech Biotech Company, respectively. She even managed to obtain a Ph.D. in Public Policy from the University of Arkansas at Fayetteville, with a double specialization in Health and Leadership Policy.

Obtaining a doctorate while working full-time was an unbelievably challenging experience in itself, especially working covering a multi-state territory. To complicate matters, the University of Arkansas at Fayetteville was a roughly 3–4 hour drive (one-way) depending on traffic and construction. And since construction was going on about 90% of the five years while pursuing her Ph.D. on a part-time basis, this required her to make a roughly 8-hour round trip drive to attend her required 1–2 classes per week. But she had more to worry about then just her completing this journey, including a series of health setbacks experienced by both Terry and her.

During one particular time during a major lupus flare, Michele was hospitalized for an extended time and endured physical, mental, and emotional exhaustion. Following a moment of weariness and depression, she made the decision to drop out of her doctorate program. But since she has never been a quitter, Michele immediately felt like a failure and regretted her decision. Her academic cohorts also reached out to her and encouraged her to reconsider her decision. She remembers one of them saying, "Michele, we know you are tired and can no longer do this on your own; but rest and regroup and let's do this together." At that moment she knew what she had to do and that is what she has done all of her life—finish what she started. And that is exactly what she did and in May 2006, Michele earned her doctorate and officially became Dr. Michele Wright, Ph.D.

With advanced degrees in engineering and public policy, Michele was able to utilized her accumulative work experience to transition into her role as a multi-dimensional Senior Executive with experience providing dynamic leadership in diverse roles, including healthcare administration and business development to Fortune 100 companies and an international non-profit organization., including during her tenure as the Chief Executive Officer of the Greater Ozarks-Arkansas Region with the American Red Cross.

But one of her biggest rewards was still in the making. Not only did Michele find healing and new beginnings in Little Rock, but on November 1, 1999, she was introduced to Terry Wright via a mutual friend and blind date. It didn't take long for both to see that they were a match made in heaven, even without either knowing and understanding the realities of both of their rare and genetic diseases. Although Terry knew of Michele's lupus diagnosis and Michele knew of Terry's unnamed medical events, it didn't lessen their extreme love for one another, because they were both opened and transparent about their journey. But it would be the "in sickness and in health" that would ultimately prove the true test of "to love and to cherish, till death do us part..." For Michele and Terry would proceed on a journey that neither one of them could have envisioned nor prepared for and one that would ultimately earn Terry his purple ribbon and purple rose, in his journey to uncovering cystic fibrosis.

4 Terry Wright, African American (BIPOC) Man with Genetic Disease Cystic Fibrosis (CF)

Terry Gene Wright was born on August 16, 1962 in Little Rock, Arkansas to Rose Wright and the Late James Wright. But his numerous health issues were apparent and extreme just as his love for sports and outdoor activities.

At a very young age and as young as he can remember, Terry experienced severe stomach issues that he often describes as "being kicked in the gut by a donkey." During his countless hospitalizations, doctors concluded that Terry's gastrointestinal health challenges likely came from ulcers or under the categories of other commonly known stomach disorders. This was coupled with concerning breathing issues which were labeled as well as a bad case of asthma.

As a child, this was devastating and difficult to Terry, especially being so young and not understanding why or what was happening to him. It also made him different from other children. Because, he was the one always missing school. And when he did go to school and played, he was the one breathing hard, sweating hard, and wondering hard "Why Me?" As a consequence, he believes this impacted not only his educational outcomes but left him with a lot of physical and mental scars that he carries to this very day.

Terry often felt lonely during his many hospitalizations and medical woes. But he was introduced to two new friends, Demerol (an opioid pain medication, a.k.a., narcotic) and Phenergan (a sedative/anti-nausea medication), that would remain important associates of him for decades to come. This combination was commonly used to treat moderate to severe pain and was collectively the one thing that intermittently reduced his pain and made him feel more at ease, even if for the moment, therefore allowing him to temporality feel relief. But he would soon learn that he had two new friends on the horizon, physical fitness and sports.

Terry always was a natural born athlete, especially due to his impressive athleticism and strong performance in various sports at a young age, despite his medical challenges. This was definitely in his DNA since all of his siblings displayed some form of fitness acumen. Due to Terry's natural athletic ability and love for fitness and sports, he tried to often underplay the severity of his asthma to his parents. Consequently, he excelled and impressed in many athletic activities, starting with baseball at the age of six. Coached by his dad James, Terry and his athletic brother Tony, who were pitching, hitting home runs, and knocking balls out the park, were destined for the Major League Baseball. But in middle school, Terry decided to transition from baseball to track and field in the 6th grade. He started off with speed competitions in 5K and 10K races and runs. Terry advanced quickly and joined the relay team as the 3rd leg from 6–12th grade. He also ran the 100-yard dash, 220-yard dash, 440-yard dash (quarter-mile race), 4 × 100 m relay, and 300 meters hurdles.

At the age of 19, Terry continued his athleticism, with the launch of his career as a certified personal fitness trainer at the former French Riviera Health Spa that located in Little Rock, Arkansas. This is where Terry learned that he had a passion and talent to not only obtain excellent physical fitness but to help others achieve impressive physical conditioning as well. Seeing the array of physical and mental benefits for himself and others, he has been physical training ever since. Around the age of 22, he entered the field of martial arts where he remained faithfully for several years and where he achieved a 3rd degree black belt and won many competitions in Taekwondo. Terry's connection to the martial arts in general and Taekwondo particularly extended beyond his physical fighting skills and health improvements. This Korean traditional martial art also greatly benefited his mental health and strength, self-esteem and confidence, and overall well-being and self-discipline.

He also discovered a love for modeling in his 20's while enjoying playing tennis, racquetball, ping pong. In his 30's, he stepped up to teaching high-energy step aerobics while competing and winning numerous pickleball—defined by Wikipedia as a paddleball sport (similar to a racket sport) that combines elements of badminton, table tennis, and tennis[8]—competitions. During this same era, Terry would run and compete in 5k, 10k, marathon, and 100-mile bike competitions, while often finishing towards the top.

Terry's attitude about sports competition mirrored his philosophy about life overall: "There are no mountains too high to conquer." This was embedded in him at the age of 12 when his physical health mentor named Curtis Johnson, a war veteran with extensive training in the kung fu style of martial arts that Terry met through his older brother Tony, first took Terry up Pinnacle Mountain, the second highest natural point in Pulaski County, Arkansas and located in the foothills of the Ouachita Mountains just outside of Little Rock, according to Wikipedia.[9] Terry credits that experience to him becoming an avid mountain climber. Additionally, Curtis introduced Terry to the field of herbalism. And this early training and exposure have remained an integral part of his life and quality of being.

But even with all of this extensive physical training, strong health conditioning, and valuable herbal training, Terry had an unknown stranger lurking in his life and body. This unknown disease would continue to work havoc on his life and bring pain, suffering, and destruction in ways unimaginable. But he was destined to find a helper and soulmate as he continued growing older.

As a certified personal trainer, Terry had many clients and associates. One of his clients named Theo told him about a single available young lady named Michele Wise that he felt he should meet. Terry was cautiously optimistic but very skeptical. Nonetheless, he asked Theo to show him a photo of Michele. He told Theo that it was something about her eyes and asked him to proceed to set up what would become his first and last blind date. On November 1, 1999, Michele and Terry met and it felt like they both had found their better half. Within minutes of meeting Michele, Terry gave her the nickname "Butterbean." When Michele asked Terry why did he call her Butterbean, he said she just looked like a big juicy Butterbean. Michele accepted this nickname which would continue to follow her throughout their entire life together. But not even Butterbean was unaware of the unexpected journey ahead.

During their blind date, Terry had to make a quick run to the restroom. Michele didn't think much about it until she realized he made frequent bathroom trips on every single subsequent date as well. She would also often hear Terry in the rest room vomiting violently. Terry explained that he had a bad stomach that he had been dealing with his entire life, since he viewed his condition as an unwanted and ruthless character defect. Within the first weeks of them dating, Terry had to make several late night runs to the nearest emergency room after being severely ill all day. But he was not alone during these times. First of all, he had his Butterbean faithfully by his side throughout every trip to the hospital. He also looked forward to reconnecting with his two old and reliable friends, Demerol and Phenergan, because they never seem to fail him or his pain when he needed them most. Michele knew that something was seriously wrong with Terry while their love continued to grow stronger and stronger. Their love prevailed and they were both ready and willing to make their union official.

On November 4, 2000, Terry and Michele joined together in marriage. They both took the finer details of their vows seriously—which proved very fortunate, as the "in sickness and in health" part soon got put to the test!

Their honeymoon proved somewhat unique because Terry had to head to the emergency room because of his relentless stomach pains and uncontrollable vomiting. As much as they had hoped for normalcy, Terry being sick was his and Michele's new normal, as was the diagnosis of lupus was Michele's just almost seven years prior. But the situation only seemed to get worse and more dire.

Because of her in-depth pharmaceutical background, Michele was accustomed to the signs of pneumonia and urged Terry to go to a close by walk-in clinic when he began to show similar signs. Terry agreed.

Upon being examined, the physician advised Terry that if he were not black, he would say that he had cystic fibrosis. The conversation was quickly changed to the fact that Terry was just diagnosed with double pneumonia. However, the doctor cautiously decided to send Terry home to be treated. Terry's pneumonia prognosis eventually improved while his health continued to decline. To the point, that they sought multiple healthcare specialists including a former general surgeon in Little Rock who clearly stated that Terry had the most damaged pancreas he had ever seen in the multi-decade career. He further shared that after seeing the photos of the condition of Terry's pancreas that he was expecting to see a 90-year old man enter his office in a wheelchair. Interestingly enough, ageist biases in medicine are a reality that may often intersect with racism. But in reality, Terry entered after literally just running a few back to back marathons. Nonetheless, Terry and Michele were still desperate for answers and this well-respected surgeon was willing to try to help, because it was important to them to finally find someone who was willing and hopefully qualified to help what no one else seem to achieve.

In 2001, Terry went under the knife for what would be an 8-hour pancreaticojejunostomy (also known as the Puestow procedure), a surgical technique that is used in the treatment of chronic pancreatitis. Three years following Terry's surgery, O'Neil and Aranha (2004) noted:

> Chronic pancreatitis is a progressive fibrosis of the pancreas that leads to loss of endocrine and exocrine function. The most common symptom in this disease is intractable pain. The etiology of pain in chronic pancreatitis is not clearly understood. However, many of these patients have dilated ducts consisting of saccular dilations and intervening constructions referred to as the "chain of lakes" phenomenon. These patients can be diagnosed with either endoscopic retrograde cholangiopancreatography (ERCP) or computed tomography (CT). These patients are best treated by the Partington Rochelle modification of the Puestow Procedure otherwise known as lateral pancreaticojejunostomy. Overall pain relief in published studies occurs in 50–90% of patients. Another proposed advantage of the

> lateral pancreaticojejunostomy is preservation of endocrine and exocrine pancreatic function as long as the pancreas is not further damaged by alcohol.

Following this major procedure and a roughly one-month hospital stay, Terry was introduced to a simple but transformational therapy called pancreatic enzyme supplements. These enzymes, coupled with his surgery, helped Terry to finally experience more thorough and effective digestion by giving his body the substances needed to break food down and get absorbed through the intestinal walls. This meant that Terry could enjoy food or a meal that felt normal (a concept that Terry had admired about others in his circle most of his entire life) with his wife. This also helped to minimize Terry's concerns about eating and immediately getting very sick in public places. This resulted from his fear of embarrassment and humiliation of experiencing uncontrollable vomiting and bowels accidents that he so often experienced privately.

But over the next 16-plus years, Terry's health issues were far from over or resolved with back to back hospitalizations, surgeries, and frightening moments where the line between life and death became very narrow. The tipping point for Terry came when he was hospitalized in critical condition from Christmas of 2016 through New Year's 2017. Michele was extremely concerned that if they didn't find answers soon, then there was a good chance that Terry would not be around to see 2018.

This became all the more apparent when the hospital where Terry was admitted appeared to use everything they had at their disposal (high-powered antibiotics, antivirals, breathing apparatuses, oxygen, etc.) in an attempt to get Terry better. But his prognosis continued to worsen. This is when Michele knew the time had come for drastic action to save Terry's life." That's when her pharmaceutical background and past history of selling antibiotics proved an invaluable asset in helping Terry to get the right care.

During her tenure in pharmaceutical sales with Pfizer, Michele promoted a newly released quinolone antibiotic and called on Infectious Disease (ID) doctors to promote its broad spectrum of indications. Coming back to remembrance, Michele reflected how ID clinicians were the ones to often solve enduring mysteries preventing patients from getting accurate diagnoses for the underlying causes of recurrent infections. ID doctors usually have around 10 years of specialized training in fields like microbiology or tropical diseases.

Michele was also taken back that Terry was never referred to an ID provider for further evaluation. So, in early 2017, after Terry's release from his prolonged stay in the hospital, she decided to search out an ID clinician on her own. She decided to start with the University of Arkansas for Medical Sciences (UAMS); their status as a major research and teaching hospital meant they had extensive resources that could prove vital in getting Terry an accurate diagnosis and appropriate care. To her shock, not only did UAMS have ID's onboard but an entire Infectious Diseases Clinic.

Michele did not hesitate to make Terry the earliest available appointment possible. But this time, it would be about listening to the patients instead of the color of the patient's skin. Thus, within 30–45 minutes of listening to Terry and Michele, the ID doctor concluded that in spite of Terry being African American, he was convinced that he had the classic signs of cystic fibrosis. Unlike 17 years earlier when Terry's doctor had said "if you weren't Black," this clinician decided to at least rule out the possibility. Terry was then sent back to the same children's hospital that he knew all too well from childhood to take a sweat test, which measures the amount of chloride in his sweat. According to the Cystic Fibrosis Foundation,[10]

> If you show symptoms of cystic fibrosis or your baby has a positive newborn screen for CF, a sweat test at a CF Foundation-accredited care center can help provide a CF diagnosis by measuring the concentration of salt in a person's sweat. This painless test is the most reliable way to diagnose CF.
>
> People with CF have more chloride in their sweat than people who do not have CF.
>
> For a child who has CF, the sweat chloride test results will confirm the diagnosis by showing a high chloride level. A baby has to sweat enough to do the test. Full-term babies usually produce enough sweat by 2 weeks of age. The test should be done as soon as possible between 10 days and, at the latest, 4 weeks of age for babies who have had a positive NBS or prenatal genetic test.
>
> Typically, sweat chloride values do not change from positive to negative or negative to positive, as a person grows older. Sweat test results also do not vary when a person has a cold or other brief illness. If a sweat test is done correctly, then results that are positive will show a high chloride level.
>
> To understand what the sweat test results mean, a chloride level of:
> - Less than or equal to 29 mmol/L = CF is unlikely regardless of age
> - Between 30–59 mmol/L = CF is possible and additional testing is needed
> - Greater than or equal to 60 mmol/L = CF is likely to be diagnosed
>
> When sweat chloride test results fall between the range of 30–59 mmol/L, the sweat test is usually repeated.

The hospital—probably in disbelief themselves based on Terry's race, ethnicity, and age—repeated Terry's sweat test twice to be sure the results were accurate! The second test clearly concluded and confirmed that Terry undeniably had cystic fibrosis. Terry was 54 years old by this point. These results were subsequently sent to John Hopkins, where Terry's CF diagnosis was finalized. Clinicians at Johns Hopkins also had Terry's CFTR genes sequenced to see what specific mutations might be causing his illness. Like many other racial and ethnic minority people with CF, Terry had only rare mutations on these genes. Hence, these differences in genetics contribute to health care disparities for CF patients who are not racially white or ethnically Western/Northern European.

After a rollercoaster of pain, suffering, and diminished hope, Terry finally had a name for the disease that tormented him his whole life. Although it took an unbelievable 54 years to get a definitive diagnosis, Terry and Michele were relieved to have some concrete answers at long last. But the fact that this process took 54 years continued to disappoint and unsettle them. This is why Michele and Terry co-founded the National Organization of African Americans with Cystic Fibrosis (NOAACF), a 501(c)(3) non-profit organization with a mission to engage, educate, and raise CF awareness in the African American community and to help bring valuable resources, knowledge, empowerment, and support to CF patients, families, healthcare professionals, and the community.

Through widespread involvement, partnerships, and outreach, NOAACF's program scope is to ensure that the Cystic Fibrosis diverse community is educated, informed, and made aware of CF's existence, prevalence, and impact on underrepresented communities.

Sometimes it may be a good thing that we can age invisibly and not show visible outward signs of what we have been through. But sometimes it can also be counterproductive to mask our hidden scars, pains, and sufferings. In reality, our struggles and our triumphs contribute centrally to who we are and what we give to the world. Both visible and invisible health experiences are extremely important—and that together they are more than the sum of their parts. Therefore, it is really the process of learning to balance these experiences and engage in healing that helps us to find purpose, passion, and power in life with chronic disease—and to help others do the same.

Although Terry wanted to be an Archeologist growing up, he decided to instead pursue his early seeds and love for herbs, plants, and nature. Terry likes to plant seeds of life, love, and hope to help bring change for the better for CF patients, their families, and caretakers. He is an Arkansas dual-certified Master Gardener and Master Naturalist. He was elected the 2016 Pulaski County Master Gardner of the Year award winner and was a finalist for the 2017 Arkansas Master Gardener of the Year.

According to the University of Arkansas Research Division of Agriculture Research and Cooperative Extension Service,[11]

> As a Master Gardener you serve your community in a variety of ways, and in turn you receive training on many aspects of horticulture while making meaningful relationships and having enriching experiences. The first step is to fill out the Master Gardener Application. Send in the application to your local county Extension office and it will be forwarded to a Master Gardener program near you.
>
> As horticultural trained volunteers, Master Gardeners extend research-based information through demonstration and educational programs using horticulture best practices, strengthening communities and families throughout Arkansas.
>
> Master Gardeners serve their local community by answering questions, researching specific problems, planting educational and therapeutic gardens, providing public speakers and much more.
>
> After completing your 40-hour horticulture training you are required to complete 40 working hours and 20 learning hours during your first year. In your subsequent years you will provide only 20 working hours and 20 learning hours.

Likewise, according to the Arkansas Master Naturalists website,[12]

> Want to learn about the natural world and participate in volunteer projects that contribute to conservation in Arkansas? Classroom and field sessions led by expert naturalists and professionals in their fields will cover topics from trees to birds to geology to stream ecology. Completing the course is the first step to becoming an Arkansas Master Naturalist.
>
> As an Arkansas Master Naturalist you will have access to a wide range of volunteer activities that will help you learn more about the beautiful flora and fauna of our natural state, share your knowledge with others and spend time outdoors with a purpose that will benefit nature.

Terry also completed the 10-day, 72-hour, standard curriculum in Permaculture Design in 2018 taught by renowned permaculture instructor Chris Grataski of Stone River Design and hosted by Christ Episcopal Church in Little Rock. According to the article "What is permaculture? Design a garden that works with nature,"[13] Permaculture Design is defined by the Tenth Acre Farm as:[14]

> Permaculture design system with the official title of "permaculture" got its start in the 1970s in Australia.

> Its original meaning was a contraction of the words "permanent" + "agriculture," meaning that if we design agricultural landscapes, especially our home landscapes, in a way that improves and supports the local ecosystem, they could be life-giving for generations.
>
> Permaculture has more recently been identified as a contraction of the words "permanent" + "culture" to indicate that the design system can be applied to all aspects of designing a resilient culture, especially when indigenous methods of working with land and people are recognized and valued.
>
> However, permaculture's original application to homestead gardens and agricultural landscapes remains its most popular use.

According to Bill Mollison (1997), cofounder and father of the movement,

> Permaculture is the conscious design and maintenance of agriculturally productive ecosystems which have the diversity, stability, and resilience of natural ecosystems.
>
> I like to describe permaculture as a design approach for growing food in harmony with nature and making use of available resources.
>
> Put another way, our landscapes tell a story, and permaculture can help us read them.
>
> Permaculture is a design approach that can improve the productivity and efficiency of one's home-scale farm or garden, by mimicking how natural systems work.

The Permaculture Design program is about helping individuals cultivate their ecological imagination. The curriculum is designed to sharpen attendee's eyes to perceive the genius of wild landscapes, expose them to what it might look like to collaborate with natural patterns, and survey the range of ways humans might inhabit their creatureliness to benefit the landscapes upon which we all depend.

The course curriculum of this course is divided into thirds. The first third focused on theory—design philosophy, history of permaculture, theological considerations, and social and cultural factors. The second third focused on ecoliteracy and agroecology—from patterns of wild ecosystems, reading the landscape, and soil science, to strategies and techniques for food production, water harvesting, urban agriculture and broadacre carbon sequestration. The final third of the course focused on design process, protocols, procedures—engaging students in an abbreviated design simulation where they actually seek to work with and alongside the landscape's natural inclinations to develop an ecologically regenerative human habitat.

Terry has also been honored to formerly serve on the North Little Rock Green Committee and Commission on Environmental Efficiency becoming an advocate for the environment, sustainability, and eco-efficiency.

Terry has also become a prominent advocate and role model in the CF community. He became the real-life subject and inspiration behind the film *54 Years Late: The Terry Wright Story* (2021). He also shares his surreal journey to CF land in his children's coloring storybook *Terry's Journey to CF Land* (2021), which was listed in the top spot on BookAuthority's "8 Best New Cystic Fibrosis Books to Read in 2021." At the time of writing this chapter Terry was 58 years old, preparing to turn 59 on August 16, 2021. Upon publication of this book Terry had recently turned 62, a remarkable achievement for an adult with CF from his birth cohort. Because of both his own life-altering health challenges and his firsthand witnessing of similar struggles in the lives of others, Terry feels fully committed to utilizing his expertise to help others achieve better health and quality of life. He lives in North Little Rock, Arkansas, with his wife and Butterbean, Michele R. Wright, Ph.D. Together, Michele and Terry—as members of the general cluster of minoritized people within the society of Blacks, Indigenous, People of Color (in race, ethnicity, and heritage)—have become BIPOC advocates determined to use their experiences of invisible aging—and more specifically the wisdom, knowledge, and understanding they have developed along the way—to make a difference in the lives of others for generations to come!

5 Making a Difference Together

Michele and Terry have made it their individual and collective mission to raise awareness about their respective diseases and the kinds of disparities racial and ethnic minority patients in minoritized and socially disadvantaged Americans communities face.

Michele and Terry's work in health equity and health advocacy is already worldwide known and widespread respected. They were featured in an article titled "Tackling the misconception that cystic fibrosis is a 'White people's disease,'" written by JAMA Senior Editor Rita Rubin, MA.

The Husband-and-Wife team have achieved major educational, awareness, and support based milestones through a multitude of programs, events, and platforms through their participation in an array of conferences, roundtables, podcasts, and discussions of Health Equity and Disparities (in 2020–2021 alone) including the 2021 35th North American Cystic Fibrosis Conference (NACFC), 2021 BioMarin's Patient Advocacy Policy Initiative (PAPI) committee, 2021 CF Fighter Panel, 2021 Public Advisory Roundtable (PAR) of the American Thoracic Society (ATS) virtual roundtable "Conversation on Health Disparities," 2021 ResearchCon, 2021 "But You Look Healthy" podcast, 2021 Cystic Fibrosis Research Institute's (CFRI)'s Diversity and Inclusion Advisory Community, 2021 Bonnell Foundation: living with cystic fibrosis podcast, 2021 Cystic Fibrosis Foundation Tomorrow's Leaders "CF 101: CF in Real Life" National virtual event, 2021 Vertex Pharmaceuticals' Healthcare Disparities and Rare Diseases Panel, 2021/2020 CF Roundtable produced by the US Adult Cystic Fibrosis Association (USACFA), 2020 "ATS Patient Voices 9" published by ATS PAR, 2020 CFRI's "A Breath of Fresh Air" Virtual Gala, 2020 Bonnell Foundation Virtual "Night of Hope" Celebration, 2020 Cystic Fibrosis Foundation-Arkansas Chapter's Leadership 2020 Board meeting, 2020 NACFC, 2020 BreatheCon, 2020 Cystic Fibrosis Foundation publication of its diversity web-story, "CF Foundation Seeks Input from Communities of Color."

Terry Wright was also the recipient of the 2021 CF Star Award presented by the Cystic Fibrosis Foundation—Arkansas Chapter and the 2020 Jacoby Angel Award, the highest award presented by the U.S. Adult Cystic Fibrosis Foundation.

Additionally, in 2021, the Wrights co-founded and co-chaired the inaugural BIOMERGD (Blacks, Indigenous, and Other Minority Ethnicities with Rare and Genetic Diseases) Conference—an annual event that coincides with Rare Disease Day and Black History Month—to help increase awareness of rare diseases in minority communities by focusing on one genetic disease and one rare disease yearly. And, not surprising, the first BIOMERGD conference focused on cystic fibrosis and systemic lupus erythematosus, which has impacted NOAACF co-founders Terry Wright and Michele Wright, respectfully.

The Wrights also led the development of The Wright Cystic Fibrosis Screening Tool© to help people self-identify symptoms that *could be related to CF* as well as help medical providers identify people who may have CF, especially those who are BIPOC. Simultaneously, they launched their Advocating for Health Equity and Addressing Disparities (*AHEAD*) initiative with a mission to increase awareness of health disparities in minority and underserved communities and to introduce a successful roadmap and advancement strategies toward achieving health equity in healthcare, clinical treatment, medical diagnosis, and clinical trials across a multitude of disadvantaged populations.

Through their AHEAD initiative, Michele and Terry will help an array of organizations with educational content, assessment methods, and short- or long-term consultancy to evaluate their institutional culture and climate, set health

FIGURE 2.3
AHEAD organizational logo (© Michele Wright)[15]

equity goals, and transform the experience of patients and families from marginalized backgrounds.

The Wrights also released the movie, *54 Years Late*, a film that tells the gut-wrenching true-life story of Terry Wright's late diagnosis of cystic fibrosis at the age of 54 despite being seen by an array of healthcare practitioners, enduring countless hospitalizations and surgeries, and having all the classic symptoms of CF—a progressive and genetic disease that's often perceived to affect only the Caucasian population.

Written and directed by Michele Wright and produced by her own Butterbean Productions company, *54 Years Late* won the two top awards—Best Documentary Award and People's CF Choice Award—at the first-ever 2021 *Cystic Fibrosis Awareness Film Festival*! Additionally, *54 Years Late* has officially been accepted and a winner in numerous other 2021 film festivals—including: Best Shorts Competition (Award Winner), Amsterdam International Film Festival (Award Winner), Krimson Horyzon International Film Festival (Award Winner), Royal Society of Television & Motion Picture Awards (Award Winner), Independent Shorts Awards (Finalist), The Oaks International Film Festival (Finalist), Action on Film MegaFest 16th/17th Annual Film Festival and Writers' Competition 2020/2021 (Finalist), IndieX Film Fest (Semi-Finalist), and Social World Film Festival (Quarter-Finalist).

And as the Wrights expect many more wins in the coming weeks/months, they are planning to further partner on bringing *54 Years Late: The Terry Wright Story* to the Hollywood's big screen as a Oscar-Award winning full-length movie to further bring awareness to the concept of marginalized/invisible experiences of aging and highlight how the two of them are synergistically working intentionally to make those experiences visible.

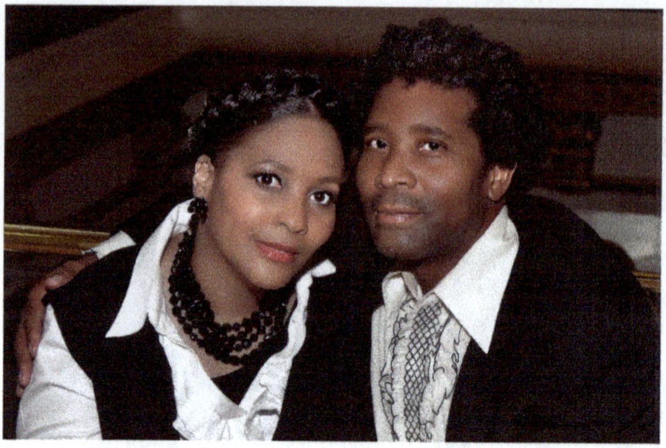

FIGURE 2.4 Dr. Michele and Terry Wright[16]

Notes

1 https://www.pulseuniform.com/coffee-time/awareness-ribbons-guide-colors-and-meanings/
2 https://www.lupus.org/
3 The purple lupus ribbon symbolizes awareness and support for those affected by lupus, a chronic autoimmune disease. This choice of color serves to unite individuals and communities in recognizing and addressing the challenges that lupus patients face nationally and globally.
4 https://www.cff.org/
5 The purple cystic fibrosis ribbon symbolizes awareness and support for those affected by cystic fibrosis, a chronic genetic disease. This choice of color serves to unite individuals and communities in recognizing and addressing the challenges that CF patients face in the United States and worldwide.
6 https://www.cdc.gov/tuskegee/timeline.htm
7 https://www.everydayhealth.com/ulcerative-colitis/treatment/weight-gain-unwanted-side-effect-prednisone-uc/
8 https://en.wikipedia.org/wiki/Pickleball
9 https://en.wikipedia.org/wiki/Pinnacle_Mountain_(Arkansas)
10 https://www.cff.org/What-is-CF/Testing/Sweat-Test/
11 https://www.uaex.uada.edu/yard-garden/master-gardeners/become-a-master-gardener.aspx
12 https://arkansasmasternaturalists.org/
13 https://s3.amazonaws.com/media.cloversites.com/f3/f360fdc4-74d7-4b81-8ad6-e086ef44528c/documents/BI_Feb_18_program_book_v1.pdf
14 https://www.tenthacrefarm.com/what-is-permaculture/
15 Advocating for Health Equity and Addressing Disparities (AHEAD) Initiative's mission is to increase awareness of health disparities in minority and underserved communities and to introduce a successful roadmap and advancement strategies toward achieving health equity in healthcare, clinical treatment, medical diagnosis, and clinical trials across a multitude of disadvantaged populations.

16 Dr. Michele and Terry Wright are the co-founders of the National Organization of African Americans with Cystic Fibrosis (NOAACF) and health advocates for underrepresented communities with rare diseases.

References

O'Neil, S. J., & Aranha, G. V. (2004). Lateral pancreaticojejunostomy for chronic pancreatitis. *World Journal of Surgery*, *28*(5), 518. https://pubmed.ncbi.nlm.nih.gov/14534819/

Mollison, B. (1997). *Permaculture: A designer's manual.* Ten Speed Publishing.

Rubin, R. (2021). Tackling the misconception that Cystic Fibrosis is a "White people's disease." *Journal of the American Medical Association* (*JAMA*), *325*(23), 2323–2410. https://jamanetwork.com/journals/jama/article-abstract/2780564

Wright, M. W. (2021). *54 years late: The Terry Wright story* [Film]. Butterbean Productions.

Wright, T. G. (2021). *Terry's Journey to CF Land.* Clovercroft Publishing Company.

CHAPTER 3

Politicizing Therapy with Older Adults Experiencing Urological Distress

Ian M. Johnson and Nicholas B. DiCarlo

Many older adults in therapy tell their practitioners that growing older is synonymous with struggle. This common statement elicits questions about the complexity and multiplicity of these struggles: Where are they located and how are they felt, experienced, and survived? Who are these difficulties to be felt with and how can one voice them? What about growing older must be suffered alone and what can be shared? This chapter reckons with these complex questions about vulnerability and marginalization.

Ageism is a "form of discrimination and prejudice, which limits the value of a person through definitions and stereotypes of old age" (Estes & DiCarlo, 2019). It is both an ideology and structural force that normalizes the experience of older age as a time of decline—processes of physical and cognitive deterioration as erosion of one's personhood. Clinical therapeutic work has the power to engage assumptions about what growing older entails and to recognize the realities of the body. The client and therapist (or "therapeutic dyad") navigate a complex matrix together of what ostensibly becomes "aging issues"—multiple and mounting physical and social difficulties, compounded losses, and economic constraints. Perceived and disclosed inequality in the therapeutic dyad threatens our ability to name and share experiences with others, feel fully seen, and play with new ways of being in the world.

Offered in the chapter are three case examples of how the experiences of disability and abjection that older people face can be politicized, demonstrating the clinical work with older adults has the potential to go beyond negotiating decline and the inevitability of death. We center our discussion of treatment around a similar impairment shared across three cases—urinary distress. We chose to focus specifically on cases in which older clients experience urinary distress because of its prevalence, psychic and interpersonal consequences, correlation with other determinants of health and well-being, and association with adversity over the life course. Through these cases, we aim to illustrate strategies for bridging emotional states with bodily realities, giving new meaning to ideas of "holding on" and "letting go."

 | DOI:10.1163/9789004708136_004

1 Literature Review

1.1 *Materialist Theories of Debility, Disability, and Visibility*

The social model of disability has critiqued defining disability as an individual impairment to prevent, cure, or rehabilitate (Berger, 2013). The social model distinguishes impairment from disability by situating it as a creation of the social, political, cultural, and spatial forces that interact with a person with an impairment (Oliver, 2004). However, the social model has been critiqued for neglecting both the embodied experiences of disabled people and the nuanced ways medical impairment and social formations of disability are intertwined (Shakespeare, 2006). Materialist theorists have asserted that the body cannot be ignored, but that a comprehensive analysis of disability cannot be limited to the body, neglecting the experience of contexts, communities, identity, and experiences across the life course (Siebers, 2012). As stated by Puar (2016), "[d]isability is not a fixed state or attribute but exists in relation to assemblages of capacity and ability, modulated across historical time, geopolitical space, institutional mandates, and discursive regimes" (p. XIV). Bodies and identities are mutually shaped through political, economic, and cultural forces (Omansky, 2011). Processes of structural violence and our relationships to structural violence shape disability (Kazemi, 2019). The gendered experiences of osteoporosis and osteoarthritis are prime examples of this convergence. Women are at higher risk for bone density and cartilage loss with limited scientific explanation as to why (Litwic et al., 2013). However, the gender disparities in the prevalence of these debilitating conditions may be rendered more legible when considering social policies that negatively affect women's health outcomes (Abramovitz, 2017), the volume of uncompensated care work performed by women (Bozalek & Hooyman, 2013), barriers to healthcare access women face (Mitra et al., 2017), and the perpetuation of diet culture and ideals of thinness that rob the body of nutrients needed to thrive in older age (Pickard, 2019).

Invisible disability has been concisely defined as "non-apparent impairment" (Evans, 2017). Impairment that is intermittent or difficult for others to detect often allows for the most options about disclosure, care and access assistance, or identity as disabled. The choice to not disclose a disabled identity or impairment can be viewed as an adaptive technique for survival, an outcome of the stigma one experiences or expects, or an act of reclamation and resistance (Evans, 2017). Materialist understandings of disability offer insight into the tensions of visibility and invisibility. Commonplace, intermittent, and covert acts of violence inflicted by institutional forces creates a process of debility across the life course. The frequency, size, and fuzziness of state-sanctioned trauma can allow it to go missing as a part of one's health and mental health contexts. Further, the lived experiences of older people experiencing multiple forces of oppression (e.g., racism, classism, ableism, transphobia) can be more easily erased and co-opted with time. For example, life expectancy discrepancies (Miller et al., 2006) and the emergence of chronic illnesses earlier in the aging process (Janssen et al., 2015) for those with mental health diagnoses are well documented. As evidenced by the landmark Kaiser Adverse Childhood Experiences study, one of the largest longitudinal investigations into how interpersonal and environmental hardships in early life extend into adulthood and later life, the feedback loop of social degradation, physical disablement, and psychological coping responses can accelerate outcomes we associate with aging and frailty (Felitti et al., 1998). Not only is state violence obscured as a debilitating force, but this violence is *embodied*, allowing the source to be made even less visible within medicalized treatment systems.

Studies and treatments that do not examine or reflect on the failures of social policy and center discussions of human rights, restorative, and anti-oppressive practices inevitably end up promoting false visions of the state's benevolence rather than grounding the welfare state's efforts in accountability. It is essential to acknowledge the ways in which health and mental health institutions exert the power to define and determine disability, assess need, and conceptualize treatment. Using medical terminology can decontextualizes symptoms, alienates individuals and communities from an understanding of illness, and advances disempowering narratives of pathology abound with preconceived notions of (dis)ability. For these reasons, we use terminology in this chapter such as "distress" over "illness" or "diagnosis" to center one's embodied experience over an externally-generated label.

2 Urological Distress

Urological distress is known as a "geriatric giant," one of the main chronic health experiences common in older age that has an impact over multiple domains of daily life (Puvill et al., 2016). Urinary incontinence becomes more prevalent in older age in all genders (Chu & Lowder, 2018). There are four types of incontinence: stress, urge, overflow, and functional. Stress incontinence is when movement or activity prompts urinary leakage. Urge incontinence refers to bladder spasms or contractions that prompt the sensation of urinary urgency. Overflow incontinence refers to an involuntary release of urine without a prior urge to urinate. Functional incontinence refers to the inability to recognize the need to urinate or locate or access a place deemed appropriate for urination. Other subtypes of incontinence include voiding insufficiency, when the bladder is not adequately able to expel urine (National Institute on Aging, 2017). This typology is not mutually exclusive, and many people experience co-occurring symptoms (Shaw & Wagg, 2017). Many forms of incontinence are either predictive of or a consequence of urinary infection (Bojd et al., 2018). Urinary tract infections (UTIs) are double in prevalence among women over 65 than they are in younger women and are most often associated with healthcare-acquired infection such as stays in the hospital or skilled nursing facility (Medina & Pino, 2019). There have also been well-evidenced associations linking urinary infection with the onset or exacerbation of neurological and psychiatric distress, including mood changes, disorientation, memory loss, and psychosis (Chae & Miller, 2015).

The dominant medical discourse depicts incontinence in a somber light it is a warning sign for a drastic decrease in quality of life over time (Pizzol et al., 2020), a predictor of other signs of "decline" among older people, such as mobility impairments (Moon et al., 2021), sexual dysfunction (Gomes et al., 2020), dementia and delirium (Bail et al., 2013), and renal dysfunction (Musso-Enz et al., 2021). While engaging in common treatments for incontinence like pelvic floor strengthening, biofeedback, timed voiding, and cognitive behavioral therapy have been evidenced to give patients greater sense of familiarity and control (Smiles et al., 2019), it seems likely people may internalize messaging that their body is faulty, leaky, and bad and something to be managed, or that incontinence is the first marker of their demise. Many of the frameworks that guide psychotherapy, too, assume that loss and universal lack are central to psychic suffering (Braidotti, 2006).

When considering urological distress from a critical materialist perspective, we think about the social construction of the distress: how it is experienced, recognized, and responded to and the relational consequences it engenders. Many older adults feel they must hide involuntary urination. When carers respond to involuntary urination, a speedy rush to reassure an individual might come across as dismissive, and a hasty intervention to direct urination to the "appropriate" place (e.g., toilet, incontinence pads) prevents any learning about how to tolerate the experience of the body's change in control. Disability theorists engaging in psychology assert the need for frameworks to celebrate the ways disabled and older people affirm their selves and bodies and resist cultural understandings of disability as loss—joy can be transgressive (Goodley & Runswick-Cole, 2013).

As practitioners, we must recognize the destabilizing nature of both acute and chronic medical events, particularly for those who associate healthcare institutions with historic cultural or personal trauma (Giesbrecht et al., 2018). Policy events, such as administration changes and subsequent shifts to laws funding and support for healthcare, housing, caregiver pay, and LTSS (Long Term Services and Supports), community-based services, what is covered in healthcare and protected in housing and community services, can replicate traumatic experiences of past institutional and interpersonal harm. The contemporary political environment and the historical life events one has survived shape how the general experiences of being sheltered or exposed to risk enters the therapeutic relationship. Laws and regulations can replicate the violations that occur on an interpersonal level; the overlap of the psychological, political, and material realities of trauma are present in clinical work. How do therapists contend with how and where we are in this landscape? Answering this question provides an opportunity for us to help patients contextualize and name experiences that are often muted by outside forces or ignored through shame and embarrassment. This chapter examines the role of psychotherapy in naming, working in and working through the hidden role of institutional violence in working with older adults with co-occurring experiences of psychic and urological distress. The aim of raising these cases we introduce in this chapter is to question the formations of aging, mental distress, and physical impairment—how are they shaped? How do they intersect? How do they obscure and/or reveal one another? What can be said about the margins of invisibility and visibility through an exploration of therapy with older adults experiencing urological distress?

3 Methods

3.1 *Type of Inquiry*

In this chapter, we present case studies of older adults who have sought mental health treatment. To locate and illustrate the embodiment of state violence against this population, our case studies focus on clients who experienced urological distress during our work together. Case studies are frequently used to provide depth in understanding a particular phenomenon (Creswell & Poth, 2016). Using this case study approach is part of a long-standing tradition in psychology. A practice-relevant case study approach is useful for informing mental health practice because it mirrors a process of analytic generalization used in treatment. Practitioners are taught to access past clinical experience and relevant theory into therapeutic interactions as the process develops, instead of imposing generalizable knowledge to formulate a predetermined trajectory for treatment (Gilgun, 1994).

According to guidelines for formulating case study research (Stake, 2006) we generated these case studies inductively through consultation and conversation with one another. The organizing presentation of urological distress was identified after discussing the topic of invisibility as it related to construction of aging and disability. In our process of helping each other reassemble and remember these cases through inquiry and idea-sharing, we also accessed our own personal archival notes as clinicians, discussed these former cases with our current consulting supervisors, and considered sources of information (e.g., documentation of historical events) to clarify how to appropriately contextualize the cases.

In presenting case study research, we have introduced the conceptual framework of materialist notions of disability, have accessed cases at various points and settings in both our careers as mental health providers, and provided contextual details that help frame these cases within the larger ecological context, particularly in understanding the relationship of the client and the work to debility at the hands of the state (Yin, 2015). Our discussion of these cases present a cross-case overview asserting tentative answers and more questions in response to the question of how the ever-shifting formations of aging, mental illness, and disability dictate what is visible and invisible in the experiences of older adults seeking mental health support.

4 Positionality

Both of us have a comfort and familiarity with the body and the role of caregiving through personal experiences of working in various capacities with aging bodies and minds. We have both engaged in care processes as hired care workers, informal caregivers with loved ones, and as therapists with older people. We both identify as queer as a description of our sexualities as well as an indication of our non-compliance with gender expectations—queerness as a social identity honors our own acts of personal and interpersonal resistance, as well as an alignment with a lineage of political dissent. This resistance is its own enactment of care for self, community, queer ancestry, and queer futurities.

Neither of us occupy the typical caregiver body as white citizens assigned male at birth. Immigrant women of color do much of the care work in the United States (Institute for Women's Policy Research, 2018). It is also immigrant women of color in formal carer roles who are treated as less valuable than family carers and are labeled as incompetent and abusive in discourse about formalized and institutionalized aging care (Boodman, 2019). Largely, our experiences as formal carers have been met with neutral confusion or positive accolade. Responses we receive—like "was that part of your training?" or "you've got such a big heart!"—conceal the realities of each of our financial necessity at precarious times in our lives, and our experiences of finding meaning in unfairly-compensated work in a feminized and racialized field of care.

Essential to our argument is acknowledging that care workers, including mental health professionals, risk ability and privilege in combating violence from the state. In our own ways, our experiences as carers are often rendered invisible in new roles—educated, clinical and scholarly roles that often represent power in systems of violence. These stories are told from our perspectives as clinicians and carers who have embodied madness and rage, but also have the privileges that allow us to embody these roles of power within the therapeutic dyad and elsewhere. These case studies were written without client co-authorship and only come from the limits of our interpretation and perspectives, which can never fully depict the value and wisdom of others' stories or do justice to clients' pain.

5 Findings

5.1 *"Diapers Are for Babies": Infantilization as Disablement*

Ian: I met Shirley while working on an interdisciplinary home-visiting nursing and mental health team. She was in her early 70s at the time and had been living in a supportive housing program for almost thirty years, moving there at the height of the deinstitutionalization movement after long-term stays in institutional settings since adolescence. According to her case file, she had a diagnosis of schizophrenia and was believed to have an intellectual disorder, though had missed the diagnostic window that sorts children into the intellectual and development disorder service world. Throughout her tenure in supportive housing, she spent several days a week at a nearby mental health day program.

Shirley was referred to me by the day program after the social workers on staff noticed that Shirley was using the restroom frequently and urgently, and how she had had "several accidents on the furniture," according to the referral form. Staff decided that she would need to be suspended from the day program because of the disruption caused in groups and the damage caused to property. In the referral process, the day program disclosed that they have seen many of their long-term participants grow older and that they needed to promote "retirement" or "aging out" of the program because the format of the program couldn't support changing needs.

During our initial assessment, Shirley vacillated between being angry with the director of the day program and telling me she had been "bad." She vehemently refused the nurse's suggestion to be referred to a urologist or gynecologist. When I noticed an expression of fear on her face, I asked her if she was afraid of the doctor. She responded by saying "I don't like being touched." During this visit, I also asked about using incontinence pads, to which she responded by stomping her feet and flailing her arms, saying repeatedly "diapers are for babies and I'm not a baby." Her apartment was on the ground floor and had a window that overlooked the sidewalk, and she reported that she felt watched by passersby. When checking with residential staff and day program clinicians, Shirley had not presented with active psychotic symptoms in several years.

It was evident to me that Shirley's incontinence was taking away her adulthood. The experience of losing control of one's bladder may evoke memories of being a child and cultural narratives about normative development. Her refusal to seek medical care and fear of "being touched" was reflective of the inherent and possible abuse and neglect in institutionalized settings, where not getting enough touch or receiving invasive and violent touch seems a likely experience. Psychosis can be aggravated by bodily experiences, including urinary infection, and her experience of being watched by people on the sidewalk mirrored an experience of surveillance that is both reminiscent of being an infant and being institutionalized. Her refusal to embody the imagery of an infant in a diaper by wearing protective undergarments felt like an assertion of her womanhood. I could imagine and appreciate how Shirley, who had been a "ward of the state" for much of her life, may experience an urgency to assert her independence.

This same driving force of urgency, embodied in rushing to leave groups to make it to the bathroom, was what she was receiving punishment for. This punishment was something she was of two minds about—a part of her absorbing the perspective that her rebellion is bad, a part of her betrayed by her community for enacting the patterns that community living was supposed to be a resistance of. The goal of the referral wasn't just to address her urinary incontinence, but to render the intersections of her aging and psychiatric survivorship invisible.

There was a nonchalance about the onset of her medical issue and a belief that her physical decline was an inevitability of aging—whether about willingness or capacity, the program was not equipped to be adaptive or enabling of health through the life course, and now that those who were "deinstitutionalized" were aging, they were preparing to discard them. Further, there was no dialogue about Shirley's life course experience or what access the day program meant to her. She had broken the rules, and there was no question or concern for how the rules were breaking her.

A social work intern I supervised began working with Shirley after our initial assessment, at first to visit weekly and socialize with Shirley, given her loss of social ties and recent breaks in trust. As a woman, the social work intern was positioned to build rapport and create safety in discussing medical issues. The interning clinician brought the idea to neutralize the association between protective undergarments and diapers by wearing them herself to a visit with Shirley. She showed Shirley the waistband of the undergarment in a conversation and explained that it can create peace of mind for adults and allow them to engage in and enjoy life activities more fully. Shirley agreed to begin wearing them, and the intern helped Shirley organize them in her clothing drawer to further separate the experience of infancy from their use.

With reassurance that Shirley would not damage furniture or create a stir with other participants, she began attending the day program again, albeit on a reduced schedule. Several weeks later, our intern accompanied Shirley to a gynecologist exam, after thoroughly educating her on what to expect using pictures. Our team's nurse arranged with the doctor in advance to reduce the amount of disrobing required for examination. Through connection with treatment, Shirley's medical team discovered her incontinence was related to a benign tumor blocking her urinary tract, which she agreed to have removed.

5.2 *"The Grave Was Reaching for Me": Urine Retention as Vigilance*

Ian: Early in my tenure as a social worker in Brooklyn, I worked with a man named Sam, a working-class secular Jewish man in his 70s. He was referred to the agency by his daughter, who exasperatedly described him as incompetent at many tasks—balancing a checkbook, rationing his groceries, preparing meals, caring for himself medically, cleaning the apartment. Sam had an ex-wife and an older brother who had very limited contact with him. Sam's wife left him for another man 25 years prior, leaving their daughter as his reluctant companion and carer.

Our agency offered home visits, but Sam insisted on walking several blocks, past a cemetery, to meet at our offices. He often wore a baseball cap and striped shirt. He called me "sir" and "doctor" whenever he spoke. In addition to calling me "doctor," he perceived my first name to be Yin, and asked regularly if I was of Japanese ancestry or had been adopted into a Japanese-American family. Before he sat down in session, he first would lay down a newspaper in the chair. Throughout our early sessions, he would sit and wring his baseball hat as we talked about the regret that had filled his life. His daughter reportedly berated him over the phone and would punish him for overeating by making him go without groceries. He had a sensory experience that he was falling every time he passed the cemetery on the way to session, which he described as unique to this specific location and time, saying "the grave was reaching for me." Whenever he left, he would leave behind a sweat-soaked newspaper on his chair for me to clean up.

Early on, I asked him how he was feeling about coming to therapy, hoping it would provide an entry point into discussing the newspaper. He described being so nervous to talk that he was fearful of wetting his pants. His imagined outcome was that he would urinate and feel ashamed that I'd need to help clean up after him, and that in response, I would ban him from attending services. He would sweat so profusely that it created a manifestation of his fear, one that he ended up leaving for me to clean up.

Sam was also fearful that his physiological symptoms of anxiety—heart palpitations, excessive sweating, frequent urination—were symptoms of a medical problem. When I referred him to a social group to supplement our sessions, he experienced obsessive thoughts about the other man in the groups' recent treatment for prostate cancer, asking me regularly if I thought he had prostate cancer, too. An enlarged prostate could in fact cause urological distress, and I encouraged him to realistically assess his anxiety and take medical actions he felt necessary. In this conversation, he disclosed that he had a lifelong avoidance of doctors because he had been sexually assaulted as a young boy by a family friend and found medical exams frightening. I saw myself included in his transference toward doctors, since he continued to dub me with the credential despite my attempts to inform him otherwise. Jewish and born in the mid-1930s, Sam's associations with Japan were one of cultural trauma. Not only was he afraid that I would shame him and reject him, but he also feared on some level that I would inflict invasion or extermination. Yet, he continued to turn to me for care, in what I imagine was similar to the relationship between Sam and his daughter, a relationship that generated fear and required a wartime alertness. In his attempts to conserve food, he would reach a level of hunger that prompted him to binge. There was a similar holding pattern with his urine in session—he created wetness in his efforts to hold his bladder despite an urge to urinate. There were other fantasies about what would happen if he allowed his body to release, too; if he let go of the tension that carried him on his walk to the office and fully succumbed to his vertigo in the graveyard, he believed he would surely die. This constant vigilance seemed both incredibly isolating and distancing, prompting a cycle of avoidance and conflict with his daughter and preventing Sam from developing new relationships or connecting safely with his environment.

In our work, Sam was able to relax into individual sessions and develop relationships in the therapeutic group. He got a referral to a doctor from a woman in his group who had shared sexual assault as part of her experience surviving the Holocaust. The doctor was a quite tender geriatric specialist, and her gender presentation eased Sam's fears. She ruled out prostate cancer and prescribed Sam a beta-blocker for blood pressure that had ancillary effects of reducing his anxiety. I allowed him to use the newspaper as a buffer between him and his seat, but also encouraged him to dispose of it himself. This allowed for the newspaper to become a symbolic object in Sam's treatment, through which he could observe the declining severity of his anxiety through the gradual decrease in wetness. Through other Jewish people in the therapeutic group, Sam began to verbalize a more politicized identity, in which he discussed his failed pursuits of the American Dream, his attachment to an expression of masculinity that he could never manifest, and the fear he felt and took on from his family and community about pervasive anti-Semitism. We engaged in a process of re-telling his personal narrative, in which Sam realized that the self-hatred and fear he had lived with his entire life was inherited, and not generated by his unique individual failings. In frequently addressing his misidentification of my race and ethnicity, we were also able to discuss how anger and blame is misplaced in a political sense. This created a space for him to begin undoing his own fear of and racism toward Asian people and created an allegory for his relationship with his daughter. I referred Sam to both a meal delivery program and a neighborhood congregate meal site to address insufficient resources contributing to the conflict with his daughter. While they continued to have a contentious relationship, the combination of therapy, medical treatment, and community referrals offset the triggers for abuse and neglect.

5.3 *"I'm So Glad You Pissed Yourself": Incontinence as Release of Obsessional Anxiety*

Nicholas: I'm reluctant to share any details about this person, who I suppose I'll call Patient X, as so much of his own conundrum in life has been trying to figure out how to show himself to others without being destroyed. He recalls hiding as a child in the drapes, full of terror. He's in his seventies now, and for much of his life he had swallowed a terrible schoolyard experience that involved involuntary exposure and humiliation. That disclosure was an important turning point in our work. The Sisyphusian weight of the boulder Patient X felt condemned to tediously lug has shifted, but it's a lifetime obligation to carry the weight of what has happened to us and our people (The patient himself introduced the myth of Sisyphus, the Greek King of Corinth who after cheating death twice is condemned by Hades to forever roll a boulder up an underworld hill. Specifically, through Camus' adaptation *The Stranger*, in which a man is condemned because he does not weep for his mother's death).

In desperate early moments of our work he voiced feeling completely hollow, as if he were a shell, or had become the curtain. Embodiment came in fits and spurts. Pain was terrifying and demoralizing. He worries constantly about others seeing past the charade of what he believes is a performance of sanity. His private masochistic process escalates mostly when others are away. He seems to enjoy me watching and what he calls "diagnosing" what he does to himself. With a strange mix of subdued glee he expresses his fantasy that it makes me very sad and must be too much to watch. Really, I just try to recognize what is happening so that he has more awareness of the consequences, and after years of work I think it appropriate he hear more about the bind he places me in: watching him do these things to himself instead of reckoning with what others have done and are doing to him. And how lonely the misery is. How eager is he for company. He expressed dismay one time when he encountered me smiling on the street an hour before our session, how could I possibly relate to him?

How confusing that so many don't really know him, and how fitting with the "logic of despair," a psychic framework geared towards proving others to be failing and rejecting (Green, 1986). Winnicott (1965) elaborates on the dilemma, we all face: "It is a joy to be hidden but disaster not to be found" (p. 187). Patient X does not let himself be known out of abundant caution that others cannot withstand his internal world, except in moments where he spills over and expresses himself in ways that are indeed overwhelming to himself and others.

When he begins to know and show the depths of his despair, is he ignored or punished by himself or others? Growing up entails becoming responsible for the ways one contains and reveals themselves, and how one is held accountable for the sadistic impulses to overwhelm and the masochistic maneuvers to be in charge of the pain. Can we bring awareness to the pleasure and relief he experiences in trying to overwhelm me? He really does care. He weeps a few times into our third year of work when I see his sweetness, but now in our sixth year and in the midst of so much in our world being difficult and worsening—anxieties and contempt for the limits are brewing strong.

The disclosure about the urinary incontinence came after an enjoyable gathering with his family after much pandemic-driven separation and isolation. He had forgotten to go to the bathroom. He was almost home. He was blindsided. The release of urine—incontinence—was a moment where the loss of control coincided with the patient lowering his defenses and enjoying himself. He forgot to manage himself with the usual obsessional anxiety about "behaving normally" and relaxed into the enjoyment of community with friends and family. He was having such a good time, he forgot to use the bathroom. He felt embarrassed, yet also felt some strength in being able to relate the episode to his clinician. He had considered swallowing the episode. I felt a flood, no pun intended, of associations about letting go. The important reality that relating is messy and that to contain ourselves so rigidly comes at quite a loss of the self. On the other hand, I see how afraid he is to lose control in a world which frames his aging body as failing, not just changing in its capacity, but failing to meet its obligation to perform. We can only imagine how the sadistic schoolyard would have responded to an unexpected, public emission.

6 Discussion

These three clinical vignettes demonstrate the range and variability of what urinary distress embodies and symbolizes. Medical events invariably destabilize psychic realities—not only can they call into question the integrity and reliability of one's own ability to contain and filter their own experiences, but they also can alter the availability of dependable and reliable others. This destabilization can bring up attachment traumas, concerns about one's survival or preservation of self, and new contact with parts of one's existential experience that has been protectively avoided, denied, and projected in the past (Kristeva, 1982).

However, approaching crisis and death can also have a clarifying focus of needing to be real, using the vulnerability as an opportunity to mourn and make meaning. There is a freeing potential realized in putting language to what's never spoken—things we don't have words for until we have work for the words to do. One way to see the therapist's role is to provide space for discovering the multiplicity of what a word means, not collapsing or forcing an interpretation, but instead holding deep appreciation for what is said and cannot yet be said. A therapist can proffer authentic responses and working theories, but a great deal of one's experience as a clinician is privately musing or engaging in our own linguistic explorations with supervisors or peers, so as not to burden the client without invitation or consent. The cases presented also offer a caveat—that our holding patterns can become dangerous when informed by our structural and interpersonal traumas, another retention that can cause infection.

There are lineages of psychoanalysis that makes the medical and the bodily a symbol and a symbol only. However, encouraging people to have a narrative sense of their bodies is an essential part of clinical work. As psychotherapists, we also tasked with considering how impairment or disability can materialize through neuropsychological responses; for example, evacuating the bladder before leaving the house out of habit or routine dread that one will not find a bathroom can prompt the bladder and pelvic floor musculature to forget its capacities and increase the risk of developing or worsening urge incontinence. Therapeutic subfields on trauma have led the charge in acknowledging that the physical sensations, experiences, and pain we can experience is a result of our personal experiences and experiences of our family lineage and communities (Rothschild, 2000; van der Kolk, 2014). Counter to a medical model, somatic and embodied approaches encourage relating to these sensations as worthy of attention, informative, and even functional. This body of literature historically has not explicitly recognized the associations between structural forms of disablement and embodied affective experience, though a growing number of psychotherapists engage with structural marginalization in their somatic work with trauma (Kidron, 2012; Linklater, 2014; Menakem, 2017). This chapter adds to this lineage by encouraging therapists to relate to the body as an ever-changing sociopolitical artifact.

Too routinely written off as a kooky old lady, Shirley's case illustrates how the societal and interpersonal expectations placed on her due to her disability predicates her failure to find a place in this world. The logic of the carceral state is that one's value is determined by labor and obedience to hierarchy. In the U.S. and throughout much of the world, big business and government colludes in creating social policy where workers are used for their labor, exploited through precarity, and then discarded when there is no more labor to extract (Gross, 1980; Estes & DiCarlo, 2019; Estes, Yeh, & DiCarlo, 2021). There is little room for the perceived waste generated from bodies and minds that are non-compliant with the needs of the state, so it was fitting for her urine to take on such significance. She faced "aging out" of the program for causing property damage. Urine becomes a dangerous and damaging thing that must be managed. Her late diagnosis of the tumor was a consistent theme throughout her life. Receiving a timely diagnosis is one requirement of many in the gauntlet of disability certification and can offer individuals limited but crucial opportunities to apply for disability benefits and programs. If she had been identified with an intellectual or developmental disability before early adulthood, she would've had access to a different, richer set of resources that could've prevented or reduced her time in institutions. Her urinary distress was a perpetuation of a cycle of neglect, confinement, and expulsion present throughout her personal history.

Sam received services due to others' concern over his ability to manage what are called "activities of daily living." Even though services were primed to come to him, Sam advocated for himself to be in the world, even if it meant exposing himself to the evocative clutches of death in his walk through the graveyard. Struggling with financial management should be a political event for any working-class person, and the retaliatory act of withholding groceries to punish over-eating speaks to his lack of autonomy, a lack of respect, and an abusive articulation of control. Even without the event of incontinence, the newspaper became a representation of his anxiety. Being present in his body and with a fuller set of his sensations assumed a risk that he would be punished or intruded upon. Through careful, curious questions inviting him to not carry this anxiety alone, a path of words more substantial than the newspaper led Sam to explore the impact of growing up experiencing sexual trauma and bearing witness to cultural violence. Sam had previously never found an opportunity to politicize his identity, buying into nationalist fantasies and fear of an Asian Other. The lack of supports he faced in developing a critical social consciousness magnified his isolation from care resources and disrupted his relationships with a diverse local community. The constant vigilance to keep oneself separate from death or harm is perhaps the same vigilance that robs us of our vitality and mutuality.

Whereas Shirley may have needed to assert her adulthood, Patient X may have needed to make contact with a more infant experience. There was relief in the therapeutic dyad as it became possible for him to genuinely lose control and experience care. The experience of incontinence came at a chapter in his work where he had noticed babies in the world being held and expressed his own longing and concern for getting enough.

The work with patient X also included naming racialized objects and processing political terror, past and present; but these feel too potentially identifying and exposing to name explicitly. On one level this is part of the transference of hiding, but there's a reality that such details increase the risks of this vignette being potentially identifying. However, it is important to allude to them as they are relevant to how sadism and control have asserted themselves as paradigms of mastery and domination. These hegemonic and oppressive realities relate strongly to how I sense the patient experiences the degradation and precarity of aging in our society. Alongside these, and again without going into specifics, are family factors of illness, immigration, chronic mental duress, and premature traumatic death that inform the patient's level of terror, flightiness, and greater contextualize his lack of exposure to aging and dying as understandable events, able to be processed and made meaning with, rather than terrifying realities to avoid.

7 Conclusion

Relational care, psychotherapy included, primes us to see and be seen with more depth. However, the politicization of the body and of aging and disability processes is largely absent from psychotherapeutic discourse, an erasure that deeply complicates our capacity to construct and sustain healing relationships. Through case examples of older clients who have faced urological distress, this chapter urges clinicians and carers to hold the complexities of patients' social identities—we must allow individuals to have their own holistic personal understandings of aging without dictating care or medicalizing experiences, while simultaneously working to name and describe disability as an outcome of structural violence across the life course and the continued inequities that prevent adequate care. When we as service providers collaborate with older patients to provide care centered around their identified needs, we must also consider the symbolic and material value of bringing the historical, political body into our work to facilitate security, connection, and agency that counter dominant narratives of aging.

References

Abramovitz, M. (2017). *Regulating the lives of women: Social welfare policy from colonial times to the present.* Routledge.

Bail, K., Berry, H., Grealish, L., Draper, B., Karmel, R., Gibson, D., & Peut, A. (2013). Potentially preventable complications of urinary tract infections, pressure areas, pneumonia, and delirium in hospitalised dementia patients: retrospective cohort study. *BMJ Open, 3*(6). http://dx.doi.org/10.1136/bmjopen-2013-002770

Berger, R. J. (2013). *Introducing disability studies.* Lynne Reiner Publishers. https://ebookcentral.proquest.com/lib/washington/detail.action?docID=6385011

Bojd, S., Soleimani, G., Teimouri, A., & Aflakian, N. (2018). Urinary infection recurrence and its related factors in urinary tract infection. *International Journal of Infection, 5*(2). https://doi.org/10.5812/iji.64903

Boodman, E. (2019). Nursing home abolition: Prisons and the institutionalization of older adult care. *Journal of Ethical Urban Living* 2(1), 1–21.

Bozalek, V., & Hooyman, N. R. (2012). Ageing and intergenerational care: Critical/political ethics of care and feminist gerontology perspectives. *Agenda, 26*(4), 37–47. https://doi.org/10.1080/10130950.2012.755378

Braidotti, R. (2006). Affirming the affirmative: On nomadic affectivity. *Rhizomes* 1, 1–12. www.rhizomes.net/issue11/braidotti.html

Chae, J. H. J., & Miller, B. J. (2015). Beyond Urinary Tract Infections (UTIs) and delirium: A systematic review of UTIs and neuropsychiatric disorders. *Journal of Psychiatric Practice, 21*(6), 402–411. https://doi.org/10.1097/PRA.0000000000000105

Charmaz, K. (1983). Loss of self: A fundamental form of suffering in the chronically ill. *Sociology of Health & Illness, 5*(2), 168–195.

Chu, C. M., & Lowder, J. L. (2018). Diagnosis and treatment of urinary tract infections across age groups. *American Journal of Obstetrics and Gynecology, 219*, 40–51. https://doi.org/10.1016/j.ajog.2017.12.231

Creswell, J. W., & Poth, C. N. (2016). *Qualitative inquiry and research design: Choosing among five approaches*. Sage Publications.

Estes, C. L., & DiCarlo, N. B. (2019). The right to work and the right to retire: A political economy perspective on precarity. *Generations*, *43*(3), 29–34. https://www.jstor.org/stable/26841729

Estes, C. L., Yeh, J. C., & DiCarlo, N. B. (2021). Precarity, USA. *Generations Today*, January/February. https://generations.asaging.org/precarity-usa

Evans, H. D. (2017). Un/covering: Making disability identity legible. *Disability Studies Quarterly*, *37*(1). http://dsq-sds.org/article/view/5556/4550

Felitti, V. J., Felitti, V. J., Anda, R. F., Nordenberg, D., Williamson, D. F., Spitz, A. M., & Koss, M. P. (1998). ACE study publications May, 2009. *Medicine*, *14*, 245–258. https://doi.org/10.1016/S0749-3797(98)00017-8

Giesbrecht, M., Stajduhar, K. I., Mollison, A., Pauly, B., Reimer-Kirkham, S., McNeil, R., & Rose, C. (2018). Hospitals, clinics, and palliative care units: Place-based experiences of formal healthcare settings by people experiencing structural vulnerability at the end-of-life. *Health & Place*, *53*, 43–51. https://doi.org/10.1016/j.healthplace.2018.06.005

Gilgun, J. F. (1994). A case for case studies in social work research. *Social Work*, *39*(4), 371–380.

Gomes, T. A., de Arruda Faber, M., Botta, B., Brito, L. G. O., & Juliato, C. R. T. (2020). Severity of urinary incontinence is associated with prevalence of sexual dysfunction. *International Urogynecology Journal*, *31*(8), 1669–1674. https://doi.org/10.1007/s00192-019-04092-8

Goodley, D., & Runswick-Cole, K. (2013). The body as disability and possibility: Theorizing the 'leaking, lacking and excessive' bodies of disabled children. *Scandinavian Journal of Disability Research*, *15*(1), 1–19. https://doi.org/10.1080/15017419.2011.640410

Green, A. (1986). *On private madness*. Hogarth.

Gross, B. M. (1980). *Friendly fascism: The new face of power in America* (2nd ed.). Evans.

Hartmann, H., Hayes, J., Huber, R., Rolfse-Haase, K., & Suh, J. (2018, June 27). *Race, ethicnity, gender and economy report*. Institute for Women's Policy Research. https://iwpr.org/iwpr-issues/race-ethnicity-gender-and-economy/the-shifting-supply-and-demand-of-care-work-the-growing-role-of-people-of-color-and-immigrants/#_ftn1

Janssen, E. M., McGinty, E. E., Azrin, S. T., Juliano-Bult, D., & Daumit, G. L. (2015). Review of the evidence: Prevalence of medical conditions in the United States population with serious mental illness. *General Hospital Psychiatry*, *37*(3), 199–222. https://doi.org/10.1016/j.genhosppsych.2015.03.004

Kazemi, S. (2019). Disabling power of class and ideology: Analyzing war injury through the transnational disability theory and praxis. *Disability Studies Quarterly*, *39*(3). http://dx.doi.org/10.18061/dsq.v39i3.6496

Kidron, C. A. (2012). Breaching the wall of traumatic silence: Holocaust survivor and descendant person-object relations and the material transmission of the genocidal past. *Journal of Material Culture, 17*(1), 3–21. https://doi.org/10.1177/1359183511432989

Kristeva, J. (1982). *Powers of horror: An essay on abjection.* Columbia University Press.

Linklater, R. (2014). *Decolonizing trauma work: Indigenous stories and strategies.* Fernwood Publishing.

Litwic, A., Edwards, M. H., Dennison, E. M., & Cooper, C. (2013). Epidemiology and the burden of osteoarthritis. *British Medical Bulletin, 105*(1), 185–199, https://doi.org/10.1093/bmb/lds038

Medina, M., & Castillo-Pino, E. (2019). An introduction to the epidemiology and burden of urinary tract infections. *Therapeutic Advances in Urology, 11*(3), 3–7. https://doi.org/10.1177/1756287219832172

Menakem, R. (2017). *My grandmother's hands: Racialized trauma and the pathway to mending our hearts and bodies.* Central Recovery Press.

Mitra, M., Smith, L. D., Smeltzer, S. C., Long-Bellil, L. M., Moring, N. S., & Iezzoni, L. I. (2017). Barriers to providing maternity care to women with physical disabilities: Perspectives from health care practitioners. *Disability and Health Journal, 10*(3), 445–450. https://www.doi.org/10.1016/j.dhjo.2016.12.021

Moon, S., Chung, H. S., Kim, Y. J., Kim, S. J., Kwon, O., Lee, Y. G., Yu, J. M., & Cho, S. T. (2021). The impact of urinary incontinence on falls: A systematic review and meta-analysis. *PloS One, 16*(5). https://doi.org/10.1371/journal.pone.0251711

Miller, B. J., Paschall III, C. B., & Svendsen, D. P. (2006). Mortality and medical comorbidity among patients with serious mental illness. *Psychiatric Services, 57*(10), 1482–1487. https://ps.psychiatryonline.org/doi/pdf/10.1176/ps.2006.57.10.1482

Musso-Enz, G. M., Capalbo, O. M., González-Torres, H., Aroca-Martinez, G., & Musso, C. G. (2021). Interactions between "giants": The relationship between internal milieu disorders and frailty syndrome. In C. G. Musso, J. R. Jauregui, J. F. Macías-Núñez, & A. Covic (Eds.), *Frailty and kidney disease* (pp. 121–128). Springer. https://doi.org/10.1007/978-3-030-53529-2_9

National Institute on Aging. (2017, May 16). *Urinary incontinence in older adults.* Retrieved July 19, 2021, from https://www.nia.nih.gov/health/urinary-incontinence-older-adults

Nunes, E. F. C., Sampaio, L. M. M., Biasotto-Gonzalez, D. A., dos Reis Nagano, R. C., Lucareli, P. R. G., & Politti, F. (2019). Biofeedback for pelvic floor muscle training in women with stress urinary incontinence: A systematic review with meta-analysis. *Physiotherapy, 105*(1), 10–23. https://doi.org/10.1016/j.physio.2018.07.012

Oliver, M. (1990). The individual and social model of disability. In M. Oliver (Ed.), *The politics of disablement.* MacMillan.

Omansky, B. (2011). Borderlands in a political economy. In C. G. Musso, J. R. Jauregui, J. F. Macías-Núñez, & A. Covic (Eds.), *Borderlands of blindness.* Lynne Reiner Publishers.

Pickard, S. (2019). Femininity and frailty through the life course. In S. Pickard & J. Robinson (Eds.), *Ageing, the body and the gender regime* (pp. 167–183). Routledge.

Pizzol, D., Demurtas, J., Celotto, S., Maggi, S., Smith, L., Angiolelli, G., Trott, M. Yang, L., & Veronese, N. (2020). Urinary incontinence and quality of life: A systematic review and meta-analysis. *Aging Clinical and Experimental Research*, 1–11. https://doi.org/10.1007/s40520-020-01712-y

Puar, J. K. (2017). *The right to maim.* Duke University Press.

Puvill, T., Lindenberg, J., Gussekloo, J., de Craen, A. J., Slaets, J. P., & Westendorp, R. G. (2016). Associations of various health-ratings with geriatric giants, mortality and life satisfaction in older people. *PLoS One*, *11*(9), e0163499. https://doi.org/10.1371/journal.pone.0163499

Rothschild, B. (2000). *The body remembers: The psychophysiology of trauma and trauma treatment.* Norton.

Shakespeare, T. (2006). The social model of disability. *The Disability Studies Reader*, 2, 197–204.

Shaw, C., & Wagg, A. (2017). Urinary incontinence in older adults. *Medicine*, *45*(1), 23–27. https://doi.org/10.1016/j.mpmed.2016.10.001

Smiles, F. B., Mazzei, L. G., Lopes, L. C., Barberato-Filho, S., Castro, J., Castro, A., Marengo, L., & Bergamaschi, C. C. (2019). Critical appraisal of clinical practice guidelines for treatment of urinary incontinence: Protocol for a systematic review. *Medicine*, *98*(33). https://doi.org/10.1097/MD.0000000000016698

Stake, R. E. (2006). *Multiple case study analysis.* Guilford Press.

Van der Kolk, B. (2015). *The body keeps the score: Brain, mind and body in the healing of trauma.* Penguin.

White, M., Wijaya, M., White, M. K., & Epston, D. (1990). *Narrative means to therapeutic ends.* WW Norton & Company.

Winnicott, D. W. (1965). Communicating and not communicating leading to a study of certain opposites. In D. W. Winnicott (Ed.). *The maturational processes and the facilitating environment: Studies in the theory of emotional development.* International Universities.

Yin, R. K. (2015). *Case study research: Design and methods* (5th ed.). Sage.

CHAPTER 4

Gender Diverse Aging

Nat Jones

When asked about writing a chapter for this book in July 2020, I initially wondered what I, a 24-year-old, could possibly bring to the table regarding the disparities of aging populations. I had only just completed my second year of medical school and had yet to even begin my clinical rotations. Surely others with more life experience would be better suited to reflecting on and expanding knowledge of issues associated with growing older than I? Nevertheless, as a young trans researcher who had entered the field of medicine with the hope of reducing health disparities for trans patients, I thought I might as well try my hand at offering some insight on the topic of transgender and gender diverse aging.

Rather than immediately diving into a standard literature review on the subject, as I was tempted to do following the publication of my narrative review on transgender biospecimen collection strategies just a few months prior, I decided to try a new tactic—reflection. Maybe this was influenced by my longest ever continuous therapy streak of seven whole months, but I felt like this task could be a great opportunity for me to reflect on my internal schemas, biases, and ideas for positive change. I did not want this chapter to be rushed or cobbled together, but rather a glimpse into current research on transgender aging as reflected in the context of my own life experiences.

Just a few weeks later, I began my third year of medical school. At my school, as with most M.D. programs, the third year is considered the most important, stressful, and memorable of the four years. Thrust headfirst into the realm of clinical patient care, third-years must rotate through all the major medical specialties, sometimes spending as much as 60 hours a week at the hospital in addition to preparing for board examinations. Third year ultimately culminates in the selection of a specialty and preparation for the residency interview season of fourth year.

As such, it may have seemed a poor idea for me to spend my few moments of off-time during third year reflecting on the trans aging experience. Indeed, medical student burnout is real, even without the added stress of wearing a mask and goggles all day in the midst of a global pandemic. The reason I committed to this project is that, truthfully, I needed it.

I had spent the first two years of medical school so buried in lectures, flashcards, and examinations that I had lost touch not only with my reason for

 | DOI:10.1163/9789004708136_005

entering medicine in the first place, but also my trans community. This was only compounded by the rigor of spring 2020, where I studied endlessly for a USMLE Step 1 exam that had no guarantee of actually occurring due to the rapidly spreading coronavirus. I had not worn anything other than sweatpants in months and felt more gender dysphoria than ever. I had no inkling of what specialty I wanted to pursue, despite needing to reach a decision in less than a year.

I had essentially spent two years of my life in a state of non-reflection, which manifested in the form of identity stagnation. If I were to continue along this trajectory, I saw myself becoming burnt-out, jaded, and suppressive of my gender expression as an older adult. I therefore view this project as my recommitment to the cause of making life better for my transgender and gender diverse siblings. By reflecting on my quarter-of-a-century of life experiences, creating a framework for exploring issues that transgender people face as we age, and searching the literature for further perspectives, I hoped to also revitalize my internal growth and charter a new, more reflective course for the post-academic chapter of my adult life.

1 Medical Mistreatment

Many transgender and gender diverse individuals are bound by common experiences of medical mistreatment. This mistreatment can take the form of not only outright discrimination, but also ignorance and indifference. According to a 2011 national report on transgender discrimination, 50% of respondents reported having to educate their providers about transgender health, 28% experienced harassment in medical settings, and 19% were refused care due to their gender identities (Grant et al., 2011).

I first noticed this common thread during my undergraduate education, where I made many trans friends through the Queer Student Union at my university. Because of my interest in medicine, many of my friends confided their medical struggles to me. One of my transfeminine friends reported being denied hormone therapy because she did not remember playing with dolls in her childhood, and was thus deemed "not trans enough" by her provider. My transmasculine friends almost ubiquitously stopped going to OB-GYNs after coming out, telling me of their fears of being misgendered by staff at uncomfortably named "Women's Clinics" and feeling unsafe in such lobbies.

Most discomforting of all were experiences reported by my non-binary friends, as they usually struck a chord of familiarity with my own medical experiences. Whenever I have gathered the courage to come out to a medical provider, an action that has occurred exactly twice, I have not received the warmest of responses to my non-binary identity. Among my friends' stories of coming out in medical settings, there were recurring themes of providers reacting with mild confusion at best and outright harassment at worst. One of my friends was told that they had to pick either male or female, and that there was "no such thing" as non-binary identities. They took this advice to heart, developing clinical depression as they tried to live as a binary trans person for years afterward.

Considering the cumulative effects of such medical mistreatment, it is no surprise that trans individuals commonly become apprehensive and distrustful of the medical system as we age. This distrust leads to increased social isolation, delayed care-seeking, and overall poor health outcomes later in life (Kimmel, Rose, & David, 2006). In a 2011 survey of transgender individuals aged 50–95, one-third of respondents reported being in poor physical health, with significantly higher rates of disability and depression than cisgender counterparts (Fredriksen-Goldsen et al., 2011; Kimmel et al., 2006). Importantly, the effect of gender identity itself is not thought to be a significant mediator in these poor outcomes, but rather social determinants such as financial barriers, fear of medical spaces, lack of physical activity, poor social support, and concealment of gender identity (Fredriksen-Goldsen et al., 2014).

Another contributor to these poor outcomes is a lack of primary care, as evidenced by one-third of transgender individuals surveyed in a 2005 study having no primary care doctor (Kenagy, 2005). This is many times the result of financial constraints or lack of insurance (Fredriksen-Goldsen et al., 2011; Grant et al., 2011). Over time, such a lack of primary care leads to decreased prevention and screening interventions, the development and subsequent poor management of chronic health conditions, and reliance on emergency departments for care (Blewett, Johnson, Lee, & Scal, 2008; Grant et al., 2011).

The effects of racial marginalization further mediate these relationships, with Latinx, Black, and Indigenous transgender individuals reporting higher rates of unequal care and physical assault in medical settings alongside poorer health outcomes (Grant et al., 2011). Unfortunately, there are few studies that take an intersectional approach to understanding transgender aging, with only a handful of studies examining the complex interplay of interrelated factors such as ethnicity, class, education, and socioeconomic status (Chen, McLaren, Jones, & Shams, 2020). This interconnectedness is especially apparent when examining trans elders living with HIV/AIDS; factors such as sex work history, sexual assault, and race must be considered in order to understand why the current rate of HIV infection is 4.28% among trans women and how to better meet the social needs of HIV-positive trans elders (AIDS Epidemic Update, 2007; Cahill & Valadez, 2013).

A host of other concerns arises when one considers end-of-life care for transgender individuals, who are poorly served by traditional end-of-life social services and are less likely have a will or appointed healthcare proxy than cisgender counterparts (de Vries et al., 2019; Kcomt & Gorey, 2017). In a 2014 survey of nearly 2,000 elderly transgender adults, many indicated they would rather die at home than in a palliative care facility or nursing home, citing fear of abuse, stigma, being denied painkillers, and having their identities be disrespected in their last moments (Witten, 2014). Although recommendations have been instituted to address these very real concerns, it is uncertain whether facilities are truly following these new guidelines, and the fear of aging while trans in such a potentially hazardous situation persists (Auldridge, Tamar-Mattis, Kennedy, Ames, & Tobin, 2012; Chin, Chiplin, Dayton, & Rowen, 2010).

There is also a dearth of formal research on how non-binary transgender individuals interact with and are mistreated by medical systems, with most of the above statistics examining binary transgender populations. The little research on this topic that does exist is very recent, with one 2019 survey suggesting that non-binary individuals may have lower healthcare utilization, higher rates of depression, and be more likely to hazardously utilize alcohol (Reisner & Hughto, 2019). As more non-binary people age, it is imperative that these disparities continue to be elucidated as they may reveal health care needs distinct from binary transgender individuals (Nolan, Kuhner, & Dy, 2019).

As a non-binary individual who grew up in a small, Southern town, I experienced microaggressions in public on an hourly basis, at best. When I would present in a feminine fashion, I would feel immense discomfort when called "ma'am" by customer service workers, who were usually just trying to be polite. If I dressed in a masculine fashion, I was constantly aware of judgmental stares and would experience the ultimate horror of "Sir—oh wait, I mean MA'AM! I am so sorry, of course you are a woman!" I endured this for four years in undergrad, and when I moved to Tampa for medical school things were only marginally better.

In clinical rotations, I decided it was easier to buckle down and barricade myself against the tide of microaggressions and misgendering I experienced from nurses, residents, and other hospital staff than it would have been to wear a they/them button and experience outright transphobia on a regular basis. This was obviously not an ideal path to take—one I pursued only because I feared negative clerkship evaluations that could potentially affect my grades. I witnessed offensive jokes be made about my trans patients. I got odd looks when I didn't laugh as my attending joked, "Oh, sorry, did I *assume* your gender?" after a mandatory inclusivity training. I was called "girl" and "ma'am" dozens of times daily.

These microaggressions add up over time, and have been shown be more frequent for non-binary populations in areas without anti-discrimination policies such as the South (Gartner & Sterzing, 2018). The fact that I, a future health care provider, experienced such discrimination from my colleagues begs the question: just how much harm is being done to trans and gender diverse patients in my community?

As I research the ways aging transgender individuals interact with health systems, I am filled with sadness that medical mistreatment is such a potent commonality among trans individuals that it is shared across all stages of life. When I was an undergraduate student, it seemed that this was just a temporary problem, one that could go away if I decided to medically transition and pass as a binary cis man, or if I were to move out of the South. Instead, it is apparent that this problem unites us much more than I had thought.

2 Gender-Affirming Interventions and Satisfaction

Hormone therapy is something I have contemplated for the past six years of my life. In my senior year of high school, I experimented with masculine clothing and square jawline contouring from the privacy of my bedroom. As a freshman in college, the friends I made through the Queer Student Union inspired me to "beta test" a new name and pronouns, which eventually evolved into my current non-binary identity. The term "non-binary" is perfectly suited to my shifting gender identity, which can be described as bigender at some times and agender at others, while almost never being fully masculine or feminine. I also found "genderfluid" to imply too rapid of gender flux, which contrasted with my subtler, more gradual shifts over weeks to months.

As my friends began hormone therapy and pursued gender-affirming procedures, I felt somewhat pressured to begin hormone therapy myself. I explored YouTube transformation videos and listened to audio recordings of trans men over months of testosterone therapy to try and understand if this was something I wanted for myself. While the idea of a deeper voice and more masculine muscle distribution appealed to me, I was not interested in permanent facial hair or any genital changes. I decided that testosterone hormone therapy was not something that would satisfy me in the long-term.

My decision faltered when I later came across the concept of low-dose testosterone. Although this treatment is referred to by many as a "partial transition," such terminology only propagates the gender binary and erases satisfaction that non-binary people may feel at other points along the gender spectrum. I was intrigued by some accounts on the internet of AFAB non-binary people finding satisfaction with a brief course of testosterone, stopping after they achieved a deep enough voice or enough stubble to affirm their gender expression. This seemed appealing to me, but as a college student in the South I had no idea where to begin seeking such treatment. I was also afraid that if I were to begin such a treatment, I would accidentally go "too far," and be forever regretful of my overly masculinized appearance. So, I pushed the idea away and tried to forget about it.

Four years later in medical school, I was excited to learn about the intricacies of hormone therapy and gender-affirming surgeries from a health insider perspective. I thought that maybe I would learn enough to feel confident about pursuing a low-dose testosterone regimen myself.

Our first lecture on the subject was massively underwhelming, providing only a brief overview of the most basic of gender-affirming interventions. Eager to learn more, I approached the lecturer, who is regarded as an expert physician in LGBTQ+ health, and asked her about low-dose testosterone. However, she had never heard of customized interventions for non-binary people and ended up suggesting Clomid to me, saying that it could potentially masculinize while preserving fertility. I was shocked at this blatant lack of awareness, and became frustrated when a brief search of the literature revealed no evidence that Clomid could actually work as a masculinizing agent.

That a health care provider known for working with LGBTQ+ patients reacted with such confusion to my question truly baffled me. I had expected such a response from someone unfamiliar with the trans and gender diverse community, but I thought I had finally found an expert on the subject.

Another two years passed with barely a mention of gender-affirming interventions in my classes, until the first semester of my third year of medical school. This lecture, given by a cisgender individual, suggested that transgender individuals may be "overtreated" and that the medical field should consider rolling back access to gender-affirming interventions to avoid regretful transitions. This scathing comment on the therapies I so greatly desired, and that so many of my friends were denied, brought me to tears. I ended up communicating with the course director about the harms this comment could propagate if it were the only perspective offered to a future generation of doctors.

What we should have been taught, is that there is strong evidence to suggest that timely gender-affirming interventions is a crucial tool for improving mental health outcomes in transgender individuals, including decreased depression and anxiety as well as improved body satisfaction and self-esteem in both the short- and long-term (Fisher et al., 2014; Nguyen et al., 2018; Owen-Smith et al., 2018; Smith, Van Goozen, Kuiper, & Cohen-Kettenis, 2005). I have seen these effects firsthand in my friends who have begun hormone therapy and undergone surgical interventions—the confidence and happiness they exude as their bodies change to fit their desired presentations is undeniable.

There are few studies that examine how gender-affirming interventions affect health outcomes in older transgender populations, but the ones that exist indicate similar outcomes of improved reported quality of life and decreased psychopathologies (Bouman et al., 2016; Fredriksen-Goldsen, Kim, Shiu, Goldsen, & Emlet, 2015; Nguyen et al., 2018). Some studies even suggest that quality of life improves more in elderly trans individuals that undergo gender-affirming interventions than in younger populations (Cai, Hughto, Reisner, Pachankis, & Levy, 2019). There is an additional theory that transgender bodily satisfaction may increase later in life due to a social phenomenon referred to as the "normal unisex of late adulthood" where older adults of both binary sexes are traditionally perceived to naturally appear more physically similar than in prior adulthood (Witten, 2002).

Regarding the safety of the gender-affirming interventions currently in use, the short-term risks are considered quite low while the long-term effects on aging populations require further study regarding potential cancer risks and adverse cardiac events (Braun et al., 2017; Dutra et al., 2019; Weinand & Safer, 2015). However, recent changes to medication regimens such as modifications to estrogen type, transdermal administration route, and dosage seem to be mitigating such adverse health events (Persson, 2009). For elderly trans populations with higher incidence of medical comorbidities, increased hematological, renal, and hepatic lab monitoring is recommended in addition to good blood sugar control in diabetic patients (Berreth, 2003; Wesp, 2017). Additionally, osteoporosis screening and prevention measures are indicated for elders who choose to discontinue hormone therapy after prior gonadectomy (Auldridge et al., 2012).

Unfortunately, the research on treatment outcomes, mental health, and bodily satisfaction is unclear for non-binary individuals of all ages, who have largely been excluded from research on the subject and lack representation in current clinical guidelines (Cocchetti, Ristori, Romani, Maggi, & Fisher, 2020).

It is well-known that most medical providers are poorly educated on how to treat transgender patients (Grant et al., 2011). That the complexities of the benefits of gender-affirming interventions were brushed over in my medical school lecture in favor of describing the sensationalized minority of individuals who de-transition or regret surgical intervention further propagates the lack of awareness of transgender health needs and paves the way for more doctors to restrict these life-saving interventions from trans patients who need them (Danker, Narayan, Bluebond-Langner, Schechter, & Berli, 2018; Slothouber, 2020). As someone who has seriously contemplated such interventions, I can attest that it is not something that most trans individuals decide to pursue on a whim.

We must instead turn the focus of our medical education to examining the long-term effects of gender-affirming interventions, encouraging students to get involved in research to increase the number of cohort studies and systematic reviews on the subject, and amplifying the voices of transgender individuals who have interacted with and been discriminated by health systems. I witnessed the latter strategy after I formally complained to my medical school about the lack of trans perspectives in our lectures, to which they responded by organizing a wonderful panel of trans patients later on in my third year that was undoubtedly the first time some of my classmates had heard such medical testimonies.

Through these strategies, we can not only circulate evidence-based recommendations among medical providers, but also personify trans narratives for those who would otherwise be ignorant of gender diverse patient perspectives. In the long term, these shifts will increase visibility of the health needs of transgender and gender diverse populations, including elders who have been rendered largely invisible in aging studies (Kimmel, 2014).

3 Mental Health

My mental health hit an all-time low in early 2020. Like many others during this time, I had ever-increasing responsibilities in the face of seemingly never-ending uncertainties. I was lucky enough to have just established care with a gender-affirming psychotherapist in January 2020, and was able to rely on her to guide me through stress-relief exercises and anxiety management skills as I studied for the USMLE Step 1. This eight-hour exam covers the foundational concepts of basic medical sciences and will be regarded by many as the most important factor in my residency applications, which made for a very mentally taxing few months as I studied alone in my apartment amidst a global pandemic and civil unrest in the United States. My virtual therapy sessions were crucial for maintaining my mental wellbeing during that tumultuous time. My anxiety has by no means gone away with therapy, but I have made huge strides in my abilities to describe my emotions, identify maladaptive thought patterns, and reflect on my actions.

My experience with mental health care during the pandemic is not congruent with what most transgender and gender diverse people experience when seeking mental health treatment. In fact, according to a survey of local Tampa Bay transgender residents that I conducted with two of my medical school peers, 89% of respondents reported a negative experience with mental health care in the Tampa Bay area and 61% had been exposed to conversion therapy before age 18. When we analyzed the presence of current mental health symptoms using the GAD-7 and PHQ-9 screening tools, we found evidence to suggest a relationship between negative health care experiences and current mental health symptoms (Bohlmann, Dolan, Jones, & Knox, 2021). This is in line with the current understanding that the high rates of anxiety and depression in transgender and gender diverse individuals are due to cumulative discrimination and minority stress (Budge, Adelson, & Howard, 2013; Vance et al., 2010).

Regarding suicidality, 41% of respondents in the 2010 National Transgender Discrimination Survey reported having attempted suicide, with those who had experienced bullying from teachers being 59% and those surviving sexual assault being 64% (Grant et al., 2011). Given that respondents to this survey had also reported significant life stressors related to employment, housing, and family life, it is clear that discrimination in the lives of transgender and gender diverse individuals is the likely source of these poor mental health outcomes.

Of note, the rates of suicide attempts in trans elders over the age of 65 are lower than in younger trans age groups, as this is inverse to statistics of the "general population" which shows higher attempt incidence in the 65+ age group (Conwell, Van Orden, & Caine, 2011; Grant et al., 2011). This may be the result of the resilience and moderately effective coping mechanisms that transgender and gender diverse individuals develop over our lifetimes (Nuttbrock et al., 2010).

This resilience is reflected in a statement made by Lee Anne, a 64-year-old trans elder from South Carolina featured in *To Survive on This Shore*, a series of interviews and photographs of older trans adults (Dugan & Fabbre, 2019). She shares:

> You have to have a thick skin to survive in the South being transgender. Unfortunately, I know too many who don't. And most of them are young. I think that over the years, I've developed this thick skin because it's either that or die. I actually considered suicide twice. I came very close both times. I remember one time when this feeling came over me that just said, "No. Be who you are." And so I didn't go through with it. I also find that I've become more empowered the older I get.

Although Lee Anne shared that she had considered suicide in the past, her statement reflects a hardened resilience developed over years of discrimination. She also touches on her experience of younger trans adults having less of this resilience, indicating a need for further support for these vulnerable individuals.

Factors found associated with better mental health outcomes in older trans adults include physical activity, leisure activity, social network size, and substance non-use (Fredriksen-Goldsen et al., 2015). Of note, religion has been shown to be a positive factor on long-term mental health in aging trans populations, although research in this domain was hindered by the use of Judeo-Christian-Islamic survey instruments which failed to adequately capture the non-traditional nature of trans religiosity (Kidd & Witten, 2008).

Regardless of the observed trend of apparent improved mental health symptomatology in older trans adults when compared to younger trans populations, trans elders nonetheless have a higher burden of anxiety, depression, victimization, stigma, and medical comorbidities when compared to cisgender older adults (Johnson, Yarns, Abrams, Calbridge, & Sewell, 2018). Of particular concern are the suspected minority of trans elders who did not develop healthy coping mechanisms as described above and experience social isolation and extreme vulnerability as a result, thereby requiring specialized interventions from mental health providers (McCann & Brown, 2019).

Strides have been made in the field of psychotherapy in order to provide gender-affirming mental health care to trans people in all stages of life, with specific CBT techniques being modified to better suit these populations and encourage healthy coping mechanisms (Austin, Craig, & Alessi, 2017). In addition to increasing access to such supportive mental health services, we must also work towards reducing socioeconomic stress by creating accepting educational environments, increasing job security for the transgender workforce, and reducing health care costs to make progress in decreasing chronic stressors in the lives of trans individuals. Finally, the creation of trans-inclusive social environments, such as sober community and fitness spaces, will allow for the organic formation of social support between trans individuals and reduce instances of unhealthy social isolation in trans elders.

4 Transgenerationally Trans

As an eclectic pagan, I describe my faith as a "hodgepodge" of whatever I connect with spiritually; this includes aspects of Slavic paganism, Christianity, and solitary nature practice. I developed this faith in my freshman year of college after years of struggling to commit to a singular existing religion and preferring instead to believe in a variety of spiritual concepts. I now find great fulfillment in meditating in nature, attending Catholic mass, and participating in local pagan ceremonies among other religious practices.

In the winter of my undergraduate freshman year, I attended an Imbolc festival in rural North Florida. Imbolc is a Celtic festival associated with the goddess Brigid that celebrates the beginning of spring and the lengthening of days. While snacking on a veggie platter, I ended up in conversation with a worshipper of the Norse goddess Freya about her beliefs and practices. This was my first interaction with a transgender elder; it is a memory I cherish to this day and is part of the foundation of my faith as it relates to my gender identity.

It wasn't until my final semester of undergrad when I attended the 2018 Moving Trans History Forward (MTHF) Conference that I met other transgender individuals from generations older than my own. I was particularly moved by our keynote speaker, Andrea Jenkins, the first openly trans Black woman to be elected to office in the United States and who helped found the Transgender Oral History Project (Lair, 2019). I had many meaningful conversations with other older attendees and cherished the familial warmth I felt in their presence.

However, I was also discomfited by some of the elders I met at this conference, as some used outdated terminology, refused to acknowledge nonbinary genders, and sometimes even propagated transphobic rhetoric in their remarks. I had to walk out of several sessions led by elderly, white "crossdressers" because their comments seemed to fetishize my existence. I remember feeling alarmed that some of the elders in my community thought and behaved so differently from me. Other attendees who were my age felt similarly troubled by some of the elders we were supposed to be learning from.

In medical school, I was fortunate to connect with a wonderful transgender faculty member who spent decades practicing as a primary care physician. For the first time I had a mentor in the medical field who was trans, and through our conversations I began to understand some of the generational differences in experiences between us. If I had such a powerful mentor relationship before attending the MTHF Conference, perhaps I would have been more understanding of the conference's elders' perspectives as products of their lived experiences.

Indeed, when I met an elderly patient during a urology rotation who had medically transitioned and de-transitioned multiple times, I found myself more accepting of their thought process. I listened as this patient confided that after they de-transitioned the first time, they decided to undergo a second transition purely because of a comment from a friend; "You looked better as a woman." I was shocked to learn that this patient had no transgender friends—a very different life experience than the gender diversity of my own friend group. I asked if they had ever heard of genderfluid identities, and they cried as I explained the concept. They told me, "If I had heard of that when I was in my twenties, my life would probably have been very different."

There are many reasons why younger trans people may feel a disconnect with aging trans people; these may include ideological differences that alienate them from one another in conversation, physical distance as a consequence of social circles that do not overlap, and the worrisome idea that cumulative effects of violence, increased suicidality, and health issues may lead to a shorter average lifespan for transgender individuals. In his lyrical essay "Trans Grit," trans activist Cooper Lee Bombardier confronts this disconnect in the context of his own internal monologue at a trans support group, wherein he thoughtfully dissects his unconscious disdain at the seemingly minor struggles of a younger trans person compared to his own struggles a decade prior. (Bombardier, 2016)

This intergenerational disconnect is not well-represented in the literature, with research on transgender aging being scant to begin with (Institute of Medicine, 2011). There are some theories that transgender individuals undergo specific stages of identity development that may correspond with transgenerational differences (Bockting & Coleman, 2016). Some research suggests older trans individuals may have decreased internalized transnegativity compared to younger individuals, with transnegativity referring to the internalized discomfort one may have with their own transgender identity as a result of internalizing the gender norms of their society (Bockting et al., 2020; Jackman, Dolezal, & Bockting, 2018). As a result, younger trans people may feel misunderstood by and resistant to forming connections with elders. These concepts resonate with the complex transgenerational experiences I had at the MTHF Conference.

In the face of so many unknowns in the domain of transgender aging, there is at least one certainty: social support in general is a protective factor (Institute of Medicine, 2011). While more research is needed on the unique benefits of family, community, and intergenerational support, there must be an increased effort to connect transgender and gender diverse individuals from different generations (Bockting et al., 2016). This can facilitate the mutual exchange of terminology and healthy coping mechanisms, allow elderly individuals to promote generativity over stagnation, and provide necessary mentorship to younger individuals who struggle to envision their future selves.

5 Conclusion

After spending the past seven months in clinical rotations, I find myself with a more hardened perspective on trans health disparities. I have taken care of trans patients in the context of mental health issues, neurological problems, and preventative care. In nearly all these encounters, I have heard health providers misgender these patients, make fun of diverse gender identities, and belittle pronoun preferences. I have come out to only a handful of attendings, and only to those with whom I had built trust and a good working relationship to avoid receiving a negative grade evaluation. While most of them reacted appropriately, one of these attendings advised me to be cautious and consider keeping my identity a secret to avoid workplace strife in the future.

This comment really affected me. To avoid workplace strife, I should keep *my* gender expression a secret? I should continue to be misgendered constantly in the workplace for the rest of my life to make others comfortable? I now realize that a lifetime of suppressing my identity and being referred to incorrectly is not a future I want for myself. I already have mental health issues as I am now—after decades of such chronic stress I would surely come to embody the more sobering statistics I have been researching for this project; an isolated and invisible trans elder.

I have set a new goal for myself; instead of working to simply reduce health disparities for trans individuals, I want to go a step further and promote fluidity in medicine. This idea is multifaceted, with the most obvious manifestation being my very existence as a gender diverse medical provider. I hope to find a residency where I can comfortably experiment with combinations of masculine and feminine professional attire, as this would be a crucial step in determining if I would like to pursue low dose testosterone therapy. As an attending physician, I plan to sport a white coat pin with "they/them" pronouns and mentor new generations of health care providers in my later years. This will increase visibility of gender diversity in medicine and validate the existence of my trans patients in our shared medical space.

While I want to promote fluidity as far as gender itself is concerned, I also want to do so in the therapies I will offer my future patients. While I still do not know what I would like to specialize in, I do know that after getting to know my patients' life experiences I will work *with* them to synthesize solutions—whether they be gender-affirming interventions, cancer treatments, or surgical procedures.

With the goal of fluidity and openness to perspective shifts at the forefront of my mind, I will strive to accommodate the natural flux of medicine. This flux can be seen in depressive episodes that come and go, cancers that fall into remission, children that bounce back after severe sepsis, addictions that re-ignite with the glimpse of a cigarette lighter. Some patients interpret the flux associated with their chronic illnesses as interruptions in an otherwise "normal" life—interruptions that can be fleeting in situations like mild relapsing-remitting multiple sclerosis or devastating in Hodgkin's lymphomas that require multiple rounds of chemotherapy and radiation (Charmaz, 1991).

As medical providers, when we fail to accommodate fluidity and instead practice buzzword-based medicine, refuse to acknowledge other diagnoses, and indiscriminately apply cookie-cutter treatments, we lose sight of what it means to be a health care provider. This lack of fluidity is no doubt reflected in my attending's recent advice to keep my gender identity a secret in the workplace.

In the same way that everyone benefits from interventions that increase accessibility for disabled individuals, everyone will benefit from increased fluidity in medicine. People who have just been married or go by a nickname would benefit just as much as trans people from the ability to customize names in the electronic medical record. Nursing home staff trained in gender-affirming hormone therapies and surgeries will also be more comfortable assisting elderly cisgender men who may be on testosterone therapy or have penile implants. More broadly, patients with complex diagnoses requiring collaboration from multiple teams would benefit from practitioners who reflect carefully on potential interventions and accept other teams' perspectives with grace.

And as I age over the years, I hope to continue this journey of reflection by promoting fluidity within myself. I will not hide my identity from a toxic workplace, but rather find a community that wants to build on what I can offer as a non-binary physician. My commitment to my trans community has only increased after researching the disparities we face as we age, proving itself to be one of the strongest constants in my life thus far.

References

AIDS Epidemic Update. (2007). Joint United Nations Programme on HIV/AIDS (UNAIDS) and World Health Organization (WHO).

Auldridge, A., Tamar-Mattis, A., Kennedy, S., Ames, E., & Tobin, H. J. (2012). *Improving the lives of transgender older adults: Recommendations for police and practice.* National Center for Transgender Equality. https://transequality.org/issues/resources/improving-the-lives-of-transgender-older-adults-full-report

Austin, A., Craig, S. L., & Alessi, E. J. (2017). Affirmative cognitive behavior therapy with transgender and gender nonconforming adults. *Psychiatric Clinics of North America, 40*(1), 141–156. https://doi.org/10.1016/j.psc.2016.10.003

Berreth, M. E. (2003). Nursing care of transgendered older adults: Implications from the literature. *Journal of Gerontological Nursing, 29*(7), 44–49. https://doi.org/10.3928/0098-9134-20030701-09

Blewett, L. A., Johnson, P. J., Lee, B., & Scal, P. B. (2008). When a usual source of care and usual provider matter: Adult prevention and screening services. *Journal of General Internal Medicine, 23*(9), 1354–1360. https://doi.org/10.1007/s11606-008-0659-0

Bockting, W., & Coleman, E. (2016). Developmental stages of the transgender coming-out process: Toward an integrated identity. In R. Ettner, S. Monstrey, & A. E. Eyler (Eds.), *Principles of transgender medicine and surgery* (2nd ed., pp. 137–158). Routledge/Taylor & Francis Group.

Bockting, W. O., Coleman, E., Deutsch, M. B., Guillamon, A., Meyer, I., Meyer, W., ... Ettner, R. (2016). Adult development and quality of life of transgender and gender nonconforming people. *Current Opinion in Endocrinology, Diabetes, and Obesity, 23*(2), 188–197. https://doi.org/10.1097/MED.0000000000000232

Bockting, W. O., Miner, M. H., Swinburne Romine, R. E., Dolezal, C., Robinson, B. B. E., Rosser, B. R. S., & Coleman, E. (2020). The transgender identity survey: A measure of internalized transphobia. *LGBT Health, 7*(1), 15–27. https://doi.org/10.1089/lgbt.2018.0265

Bohlmann, M., Dolan, A., Jones, N. C., & Knox, B. (2021). Negative health care experiences, health care seeking behavior, and mental health in Tampa Bay Area transgender and gender non-conforming individuals. *Southern Medical Journal, 114*(6), 361–367. https://doi.org/10.14423/smj.0000000000001260

Bombardier, C. L. (2016). Trans Grit. In Z. Sharman (Ed.), *The remedy: Queer and trans voices on health and health care* (pp. 289–308). Arsenal Pulp Press.

Bouman, W. P., Claes, L., Marshall, E., Pinner, G. T., Longworth, J., Maddox, V., ... Arcelus, J. (2016). Sociodemographic variables, clinical features, and the role of preassessment cross-sex hormones in older trans people. *The Journal of Sexual Medicine, 13*(4), 711–719. https://doi.org/10.1016/j.jsxm.2016.01.009

Braun, H., Nash, R., Tangpricha, V., Brockman, J., Ward, K., & Goodman, M. (2017). Cancer in transgender people: Evidence and methodological considerations. *Epidemiologic Reviews, 39*(1), 93–107. https://doi.org/10.1093/epirev/mxw003

Budge, S. L., Adelson, J. L., & Howard, K. A. (2013). Anxiety and depression in transgender individuals: The roles of transition status, loss, social support, and coping. *Journal of Consulting and Clinical Psychology, 81*(3), 545–557. https://doi.org/10.1037/a0031774

Cahill, S., & Valadez, R. (2013). Growing older with HIV/AIDS: New public health challenges. *American Journal of Public Health, 103*(3), e7–e15. https://doi.org/10.2105/AJPH.2012.301161

Cai, X., Hughto, J. M. W., Reisner, S. L., Pachankis, J. E., & Levy, B. R. (2019). Benefit of gender-affirming medical treatment for transgender elders: Later-life alignment of mind and body. *LGBT Health, 6*(1), 34–39. https://doi.org/10.1089/lgbt.2017.0262

Charmaz, K. (1991). *Good days, bad days: The self in chronic illness and time.* Rutgers University Press.

Chen, J., McLaren, H., Jones, M., & Shams, L. (2020). The aging experiences of LGBTQ ethnic minority elders: A systematic review. *Gerontologist*. https://doi.org/10.1093/geront/gnaa134

Chin, N., Chiplin Jr., A. J., Dayton, K., & Rowen, M. (2010). Asserting choice: Health care, housing, and property—Planning for lesbian, gay, bisexual, and transgender older adults. *Clearinghouse Review Journal of Poverty Law and Policy, 43*(11–12), 522–533.

Cocchetti, C., Ristori, J., Romani, A., Maggi, M., & Fisher, A. D. (2020). Hormonal treatment strategies tailored to non-binary transgender individuals. *Journal of Clinical Medicine, 9*(6). https://doi.org/10.3390/jcm9061609

Conwell, Y., Van Orden, K., & Caine, E. D. (2011). Suicide in older adults. *The Psychiatric Clinics of North America, 34*(2), 451–468, ix. https://doi.org/10.1016/j.psc.2011.02.002

Danker, S., Narayan, S. K., Bluebond-Langner, R., Schechter, L. S., & Berli, J. U. (2018). Abstract: A survey study of surgeons' experience with regret and/or reversal of gender-confirmation surgeries. *Plastic and Reconstructive Surgery Global Open, 6*(9 Suppl), 189–189. https://doi.org/10.1097/01.GOX.0000547077.23299.00

de Vries, B., Gutman, G., Humble, A., Gahagan, J., Chamberland, L., Aubert, P., … Mock, S. (2019). End-of-life preparations among LGBT older Canadian adults: The missing conversations. *International Journal of Aging & Human Development, 88*(4), 358–379. https://doi.org/10.1177/0091415019836738

Dugan, J. T., & Fabbre, V. (2019). *To survive on this shore: Photographs and interviews with transgender and gender nonconforming older adults*. https://www.eastman.org/tsots

Dutra, E., Lee, J., Torbati, T., Garcia, M., Merz, C. N. B., & Shufelt, C. (2019). Cardiovascular implications of gender-affirming hormone treatment in the transgender population. *Maturitas, 129*, 45–49. https://doi.org/10.1016/j.maturitas.2019.08.010

Fisher, A. D., Castellini, G., Bandini, E., Casale, H., Fanni, E., Benni, L., … Rellini, A. H. (2014). Cross-sex hormonal treatment and body uneasiness in individuals with gender dysphoria. *The Journal of Sexual Medicine, 11*(3), 709–719. https://doi.org/10.1111/jsm.12413

Fredriksen-Goldsen, K. I., Cook-Daniels, L., Kim, H. J., Erosheva, E. A., Emlet, C. A., Hoy-Ellis, C. P., … Muraco, A. (2014). Physical and mental health of transgender older adults: An at-risk and underserved population. *Gerontologist, 54*(3), 488–500. https://doi.org/10.1093/geront/gnt021

Fredriksen-Goldsen, K. I., Kim, H.-J., Emlet, C. A., Muraco, A., Erosheva, E. A., Hoy-Ellis, C. P., … Petry, H. (2011). *The aging and health report: Disparities and resilience among lesbian, gay, bisexual, and transgender older adults*. Institute for Multigenerational Health.

Fredriksen-Goldsen, K. I., Kim, H. J., Shiu, C., Goldsen, J., & Emlet, C. A. (2015). Successful aging among LGBT older adults: Physical and mental health-related quality of life by age group. *Gerontologist, 55*(1), 154–168. https://doi.org/10.1093/geront/gnu081

Gartner, R. E., & Sterzing, P. R. (2018). Social ecological correlates of family-level interpersonal and environmental microaggressions toward sexual and gender minority adolescents. *Journal of Family Violence, 33*(1), 1–16. https://doi.org/10.1007/s10896-017-9937-0

Grant, J. M., Mottet, L. A., Tanis, J., Harrison, J., Herman, J. L., & Keisling, M. (2011). *Injustice at every turn: A report of the national transgender discrimination survey*. National Center for Transgender Equality and National Gay and Lesbian Task Force.

Institute of Medicine. (2011). *The health of lesbian, gay, bisexual, and transgender people: Building a foundation for better understanding*. The National Academies Press.

Jackman, K. B., Dolezal, C., & Bockting, W. O. (2018). Generational differences in internalized transnegativity and psychological distress among feminine spectrum transgender people. *LGBT Health, 5*(1), 54–60. https://doi.org/10.1089/lgbt.2017.0034

Johnson, K., Yarns, B. C., Abrams, J. M., Calbridge, L. A., & Sewell, D. D. (2018). Gay and gray session: An interdisciplinary approach to transgender aging. *The American Journal of Geriatric Psychiatry, 26*(7), 719–738. https://doi.org/10.1016/j.jagp.2018.01.208

Kcomt, L., & Gorey, K. M. (2017). End-of-life preparations among lesbian, gay, bisexual, and transgender people: Integrative review of prevalent behaviors. *Journal of Social Work in End-of-Life & Palliative Care, 13*(4), 284–301. https://doi.org/10.1080/15524256.2017.1387214

Kenagy, G. P. (2005). Transgender health: Findings from two needs assessment studies in Philadelphia. *Health and Social Work, 30*(1), 19–26. https://doi.org/10.1093/hsw/30.1.19

Kidd, J. D., & Witten, T. M. (2008). Understanding spirituality and religiosity in the transgender community: Implications for aging. *Journal of Religion, Spirituality & Aging, 20*(1–2), 29–62. https://doi.org/10.1080/15528030801922004

Kimmel, D. (2014). Lesbian, gay, bisexual, and transgender aging concerns. *Clinical Gerontologist, 37*(1), 49–63. https://doi.org/10.1080/07317115.2014.847310

Kimmel, D. C., Rose, T., & David, S. (2006). *Lesbian, gay, bisexual and transgender aging: Research and clinical perspectives*. Columbia University Press.

Lair, L. O. (2019). New York City trans oral history project The Tretter Transgender Oral History Project. *The Oral History Review, 46*(2), 430–434. https://doi.org/10.1093/ohr/ohz025

McCann, E., & Brown, M. J. (2019). The mental health needs and concerns of older people who identify as LGBTQ+: A narrative review of the international evidence. *Journal of Advanced Nursing, 75*(12), 3390–3403. https://doi.org/10.1111/jan.14193

Nguyen, H. B., Chavez, A. M., Lipner, E., Hantsoo, L., Kornfield, S. L., Davies, R. D., & Epperson, C. N. (2018). Gender-affirming hormone use in transgender individuals: Impact on behavioral health and cognition. *Current Psychiatry Reports, 20*(12), 110. https://doi.org/10.1007/s11920-018-0973-0

Nolan, I. T., Kuhner, C. J., & Dy, G. W. (2019). Demographic and temporal trends in transgender identities and gender confirming surgery. *Translational Andrology and Urology, 8*(3), 184–190. https://doi.org/10.21037/tau.2019.04.09

Nuttbrock, L., Hwahng, S., Bockting, W., Rosenblum, A., Mason, M., Macri, M., & Becker, J. (2010). Psychiatric impact of gender-related abuse across the life course of male-to-female transgender persons. *The Journal of Sex Research, 47*(1), 12–23. https://doi.org/10.1080/00224490903062258

Owen-Smith, A. A., Gerth, J., Sineath, R. C., Barzilay, J., Becerra-Culqui, T. A., Getahun, D., … Goodman, M. (2018). Association between gender confirmation treatments and perceived gender congruence, body image satisfaction, and mental health in a cohort of transgender individuals. *The Journal of Sexual Medicine, 15*(4), 591–600. https://doi.org/10.1016/j.jsxm.2018.01.017

Persson, D. I. (2009). Unique challenges of transgender aging: Implications from the literature. *Journal of Gerontological Social Work, 52*(6), 633–646.

Reisner, S. L., & Hughto, J. M. W. (2019). Comparing the health of non-binary and binary transgender adults in a statewide non-probability sample. *PLoS One, 14*(8), e0221583. https://doi.org/10.1371/journal.pone.0221583

Slothouber, V. (2020). (De)trans visibility: Moral panic in mainstream media reports on de/retransition. *European Journal of English Studies, 24*(1), 89–99. https://doi.org/10.1080/13825577.2020.1730052

Smith, Y. L., Van Goozen, S. H., Kuiper, A. J., & Cohen-Kettenis, P. T. (2005). Sex reassignment: Outcomes and predictors of treatment for adolescent and adult transsexuals. *Psychological Medicine, 35*(1), 89–99. https://doi.org/10.1017/s0033291704002776

Vance, S. R., Cohen-Kettenis, P. T., Drescher, J., Meyer-Bahlburg, H. F. L., Pfäfflin, F., & Zucker, K. J. (2010). Opinions about the DSM gender identity disorder diagnosis: Results from an international survey administered to organizations concerned with the welfare of transgender people. *International Journal of Transgenderism, 12*(1), 1–14. https://doi.org/10.1080/15532731003749087

Weinand, J. D., & Safer, J. D. (2015). Hormone therapy in transgender adults is safe with provider supervision: A review of hormone therapy sequelae for transgender individuals. *Journal of Clinical & Translational Endocrinology, 2*(2), 55–60. https://doi.org/10.1016/j.jcte.2015.02.003

Wesp, L. (2017). *Diabetes mellitus.* USCF Transgender Care and Treatment Guidelines. https://transcare.ucsf.edu/guidelines/diabetes

Witten, T. M. (2002). Geriatric care and management issues for the transgender and intersex populations. *Geriatric Care Management Journal, 12*(3), 20–24.

Witten, T. M. (2014). End of life, chronic illness, and trans-identities. *Journal of Social Work in End-of-Life & Palliative Care, 10*(1), 34–58. https://doi.org/10.1080/15524256.2013.877864

CHAPTER 5

Resilience in the Face of Life Challenges Experienced by Older Adults Living with HIV

Kristen D. Krause

1 Background: HIV/AIDS in the United States

In the United States (US), adults over the age of 50 constitute the majority of the nearly 1.1 million people living with HIV/AIDS (PLWHA) (Centers for Disease Control and Prevention, 2022). While the epidemic still disproportionally affects gay and bisexual men in the United States (US), injection drug users and heterosexual women accounted for almost one-third of new HIV diagnoses in 2020 (Centers for Disease Control and Prevention, 2022). Furthermore, there are disparities by race/ethnicity with White people only comprising 35.5% of all PLWHA in the US (Centers for Disease Control and Prevention, 2022). Older PLWHA face myriad social, physical, and mental health stressors not only related to living with HIV/AIDS, but also the aging process in general and the long-term impact of being on antiretroviral treatment (ART) (Halkitis et al., 2017).

While these statistics are high, UNAIDS reports that globally, there has been a 68% decrease in AIDS-related deaths since the peak in 2004, a 54% decrease in new HIV infections since 2010, and in 2021 88% of people who knew their status were accessing treatment with 68% of those reaching viral suppression (UNAIDS, 2022). Now that those infected with HIV/AIDS are living longer than before, there are many facets of their health that are under-researched including the long-term impact of comorbidities, polypharmacy, and chronic stressors.

In February 2019, the federal government launched a widespread 'Ending the HIV Epidemic' initiative (HIV.gov, 2022) after several states (including New York, California, New Jersey, Illinois, Colorado, Arizona among others) had implemented similar strategies. The federal initiative is built upon four key elements including: (1) diagnosing all individuals with HIV as early as possible after seroconversion (i.e., the transition from infection to the detectable presence of HIV antibodies in the blood), (2) treating HIV rapidly and effectively after diagnoses to attain sustained viral suppression, (3) protecting individuals at risk for HIV using demonstrated prevention approaches, and (4) responding

 | DOI:10.1163/9789004708136_006

rapidly to detect and respond to growing HIV clusters to prevent new infections (HIV.gov, 2022).

Federal funding was earmarked to specifically target geographic hotspots through existing programs (e.g. Ryan White HIV/AIDS Program and other federally qualified health centers (FHQCs)), utilize data to identify where HIV is spreading the most rapidly, and provide funding for the creation of a local HIV HealthForce in targeted areas (Azar, 2019). While this plan is important and a necessary step in the right direction, the drastic paradigm shift to 'ending the epidemic' may leave those who have been living with HIV/AIDS behind. In order to actually end the epidemic, it is vital these initiatives also support PLWHA (Adams & Flood, 2019). Moreover, since those aged 50 and older are now the majority of PLWHA, there is a crucial need to identify mechanisms to support this population to ensure that they not only continue to survive, but also thrive.

2 HIV/AIDS and Aging

There is a robust body of literature outlining the medical, physiological, and mental health outcomes associated with HIV/AIDS among HIV-positive adults over the age of 50 (Grov et al., 2010; Simone & Appelbaum, 2008). The loss of proper immune functioning and the biological process of aging itself, coupled with the long term immune activation due to a variety of factors, including ART-toxicity (Zicari et al., 2019), substantially increases the risk of HIV-Associated Non-AIDS (HANA) conditions (Leng & Margolick, 2015), non-AIDS-defining cancers (NADCs) (Riedel et al., 2015), and HIV-associated neurocognitive disorders (HAND) (Clifford & Ances, 2013). As the population of PLWHA continues to age, they are at higher risk for comorbidities than their HIV-negative and younger HIV-positive counterparts with more than 80% of HIV-positive people over 50 having at least one comorbidity and more than 40% having two or more comorbidities, resulting in multi-morbidities (Levin, 2012). Compared to HIV-negative individuals, PLWHA are more likely to experience accentuated aging (i.e., an increased burden of age-related damage that may remain static through time) (Justice & Tate, 2019) and have greater disparities in clinical outcomes with advancing age, such as risk of anal, lung, and liver cancers (Mahale et al., 2018). One limitation to the program of research on comorbidities among PLWHA is the variance in definitions, inclusion criteria, and measurement across studies.

It is important to highlight the potential cohort differences among those who were diagnosed with HIV/AIDS prior to and after the implementation of ART (formerly known as HAART) in 1996. Those who seroconverted prior to 1996 (pre-ART) came of age during the height of the HIV/AIDS epidemic and likely experienced myriad psychosocial burdens associated with the uncertainty about whether or not they would be the next of their social circle to die. Subsequently, many people of that cohort were confused as they continued living while they witnessed the deaths of many others living with HIV/AIDS (Robinson et al., 2008). Those living longer with HIV have been found to have a higher prevalence of co-morbidities and multimorbidities as well as poorer survival projections and immunological response than those who have been diagnosed more recently (post-ART) (Blanco et al., 2012; Guaraldi et al., 2015). Findings from one study indicate that people with a longer duration of HIV-infection show a higher probability of multimorbidity than those who seroconverted later in life (Guaraldi et al., 2015). Understanding the nuanced differences between those pre-ART and post-ART individuals can be critically important when developing interventions, policies, and programs that help support PLWHA.

In addition to the physiological co-morbidities that people living with HIV/AIDS (PLWHA) must overcome, they also face many potential psychological and social challenges. Testing positive for HIV/AIDS can yield different emotions including shock, anger, and hopelessness (Remien & Rabkin, 2001). Additionally, anxiety (Brandt et al., 2017) and depression (Bhatia & Munjal, 2014; Gonzalez et al., 2011) are serious mental health co-morbidities that PLWHA also face.

While much of the literature is focused on the biopsychosocial deficits that PLWHA face, there is an important burgeoning body of work focused on coping mechanisms and resilience in this population (Halkitis, 2013; Krause, 2020). Resilience has been suggested as one of many constructs including hardiness, grit, and coping that protect and reduce vulnerability to negative outcomes (Goldstein & Brooks, 2013). Understanding the manifestation of resilience in PLWHA will help inform interventions and policies and help to not only reduce negative influences but also to capitalize on specific resources within a community and/or population (Luthar & Cicchetti, 2000). Examining if and how resilience may act as a buffer against these stressors may lead to the development of strength-based approaches to clinical services which can have a substantial impact on the quality of life for older PLWHA. Too often, deficit-based models have dominated our approaches (Herrick et al., 2011).

3 Resilience

3.1 *Older Adults and Resilience*

Many studies of resilience have historically focused on at-risk children, adolescents, and veterans who may have prolonged exposure to trauma or other chronic stressors (Smith & Hollinger-Smith, 2015). More recently, a growing body of research has emerged examining resilience among older adults and its role in the successful aging process (MacLeod et al., 2016). While successful aging can have several components, it has been defined as freedom from disability and chronic disease as well as high mental and physical functioning (Jeste et al., 2013). Being resilient later in life has been associated with reduced levels of depression (Gooding et al., 2012; Jeste et al., 2013) and risk of mortality (Shen & Zeng, 2011) as well as increased quality of life (Hildon et al., 2010) and improved lifestyle behaviors (MacLeod et al., 2016; Netuveli & Blane, 2008).

Although studies of resilience in adults are more limited, there are many consistencies that show similar effects of protective factors to those of children (Masten & Wright, 2010). Masten and Wright (2010) outline several protective systems over the lifespan that include attachment relationships, agency and the mastery motivation system, intelligence, self-regulation, meaning making, and cultural traditions and religion. These protective systems promote resilience through setting positive goals and developing mechanisms that can help overcome negative experiences or setbacks (Masten & Wright, 2010).

In a sample of older adults suffering from chronic disease, Hassani and colleagues (2017) found that improvements in resilience were associated with a patient-centered approach after disease diagnosis. More specifically, their participants described personal experiences of resilience as an art of overcoming pain and suffering while adapting to life with chronic diseases and the process of overall senescence. Similar sentiments were highlighted by Tkatch et al. (2017) wherein participants discussed bouncing back from difficulties, losses, and challenges. Many also described illness as something they just had to deal with while also not letting it define them (Tkatch et al., 2017).

Other research indicates there are opportunities to help older adults improve resilience later in life (Resnick & Inguito, 2011). Interventions to strengthen resilience focus on improving self-efficacy, self-esteem, positive relationships, and learning to keep things in perspective (Resnick, 2018). The APA Resilience Toolkit (Comas-Diaz et al., 2004) recommends a public health approach to building resilience that involves maintaining strong relationships, becoming active in the community, maintaining hopefulness, and thinking positively—all of which can be done both at the community and individual levels (MacLeod et al., 2016).

3.2 *HIV/AIDS and Resilience*

The burgeoning literature on resilience and HIV/AIDS has begun to delineate qualities indicative of resilience that define it as a trait, outcome, or process including: self-acceptance, optimism, will to live, generativity, self-management, relational living, and independence (Emlet et al., 2011). For many older HIV-positive individuals, resilience helps them overcome life challenges including but not limited to the realities of aging with disease, ageism (Emlet, 2006), HIV-related stigma (Sayles et al., 2007), and for numerous members of the population, discrimination due to socioeconomic status or social class (Bird et al., 2004), racism (Ford et al., 2009), and sexual stigma coupled with homophobia (Herek et al., 2009). Siegel et al. (1998) conducted semi-structured interviews with older HIV-infected adults to identify their perceived advantages and disadvantages around living with HIV/AIDS. While the participants outlined several disadvantages ranging from having more frail bodies to feeling more socially isolated, they also felt like they were advantageous because they had more wisdom, they were less psychologically threatened by disability and fatigue, and that they could focus more on their own needs (Siegel et al., 1998). The maturity these participants possessed enabled them to temper their response in order to overcome negative or uncontrollable situations within the face of their diagnosis (Siegel et al., 1998).

Within the specific context of HIV-infection, De Santis and colleagues (2013) define resilience as "the process by which an individual accesses internal motivation (e.g. desire to survive) and external motivation (e.g. psychosocial support) that provide a basis for him or her to learn or manage the physical and psychological aspects of HIV infection." Once individuals living with HIV/AIDS can manage the biopsychosocial aspects of the infection, a sense of mastery starts to develop from achieving positive health outcomes and advocacy, and thus the end result is resilience (De Santis et al., 2013).

It is important to understand whether those who are resilient react to challenges through invoking processes which may mitigate the impact of adverse life circumstances on their health. Masten and Schmidtberger (2011) posit that resilience in the wake of multiple losses from the AIDS epidemic involves living in a way that does not deny the loss felt in addition to not feeling over-consumed by grief (Marion, 1996). Within the context of HIV/AIDS, becoming resilient in the face of loss and grief is a significant aspect of adapting to the changing course of the epidemic, (Masten & Schmidtberger, 2011) especially as more people infected continue to age successfully. Furthermore, Garcia-Dia and colleagues (2013) suggest that PLWHA are resilient because becoming aware of their diagnosis can be considered a traumatic event and thus coming to terms with their own mortality and potential fatality requires dynamic adaptation. Among those living with HIV/AIDS, being resilient can be viewed as the ability to be adherent with ART, reaching out and supporting others who are infected, and consciously avoiding risky behaviors (e.g. protecting sexual partners from HIV-exposure or acquiring sexually transmitted infections (STIs) (Garcia-Dia et al., 2013).

Resilience among PLWHA can also be rooted in cultural traditions expressed through spirituality/religion and personal or familial beliefs, rituals, or customs. Hussen et al. (2014) provides an in-depth depiction on the impact that religious and spiritual practices have on experiences with resilience with all their participants (n = 20) endorsing it as an important aspect of their lives. These participants, all of whom are Expert Patients, explain that while some HIV-positive individuals may face barriers to care due to spiritual practices, many patients who are undergoing counseling have integrated their faith-based and biomedical practices into their daily lives—they find ways to continue taking their medicine while fasting during religious holidays or they take it with a minimal amount of holy water (Hussen et al., 2014). Through the support of the EPTS and churches, many PLWHA in this sample felt like they received critical emotional support that helped them to overcome the negative aspects of living with HIV/AIDS (Hussen et al., 2014). Similar sentiments were shared by HIV-positive asylum seekers in the United Kingdom who described the importance of their personal faith and the belief that God will take control of things (Orton et al., 2012). Community support by way of religious or community organizations can be a powerful source of assistance and protection in times of need (Masten & Wright, 2010).

Those who credit religion and/or spirituality as the source of their resilience have many reasons for doing so outside of only prayer and worship. For example, one participant from Buttram's (2015) study explained that the outreach of his local ministry helped him secure different levels of social support that included a stable income and housing. Furthermore, members of the congregation recommended books to help him overcome his addiction problems and provided referrals to counseling services (Buttram, 2015). Similarly, De Santis and colleagues' (2013) grounded theory study found that participants who struggled with substance use and/or abuse surrendered to a higher power and used spirituality as a motivator to curtail use.

3.3 *Resilience in Older Adults Living with HIV/AIDS*

Across many health indicators, the CDC categorizes individuals 65 and older as 'older adults' however, 50 has historically been the demarcation point for being an 'older PLWHA' by the CDC (Centers for Disease Control and Prevention, 2019) and other scholars studying HIV and aging (Emlet et al., 2011; Jang et al., 2011; Owen & Catalan, 2012; Youmans et al., 2011). While limited in scope, themes of resilience have been delineated in some of the literature on older adults living with HIV/AIDS. Optimism (thinking positively) and the will to live were two themes outlined in Emlet and colleagues' (2011) work on older PLWHA. One participant in that study recalled, "it's [HIV] not really a big thing to me. I mean, I take my medicine, I go on with my life. I don't think about the AIDS anymore" (Emlet et al., 2011). Improvements in treatment options also gave participants a positive outlook: "I've noticed that the medications have improved so much that I'm not so stressful as far as being ill or dying from it as I used to be" (Emlet et al., 2011). Other participants explained that life is worth living and that they wanted to live as long as possible (Emlet et al., 2011). Similar sentiments were echoed in a different study on older HIV-positive MSM living in Quebec in that most respondents reported an appreciation for life, a positive attitude, and feeling lucky despite their HIV-diagnosis (Wallach, 2011). As PLWHA continue to age, it is imperative to build upon the exiting work on resilience in older adults so that interventions and programs can be tailored appropriately for this population.

In order to extend this body of work, we sought to examine how mental, social, and physical health is affected by resilience through the experiences of HIV treatment, psychosocial, and structural states among older PLWH living in the metropolitan area of Newark, NJ using semi-structured interviews. More specifically, we wanted to assess the potential efficacy of the resilience model for older adults proposed by Halkitis et al. (2017).

4 Methodology

4.1 *Data Collection and Procedures*

From April–June 2019, the team at the Center for Health, Identity, Behavior and Prevention Studies conducted 40 semi-structured qualitative interviews. Participants were recruited through community-based (e.g., pride events, drag shows, etc.) and venue-based (e.g., medical offices, HIV service organizations, etc.) sampling methodology. The team also utilized snowball sampling to recruit eligible people associated with other study participants. Participants were eligible if they met the following criteria: at least 50 years of age, HIV positive, reside in New Jersey, and able to travel to our research office in Newark, NJ for the interview. At the start of the session, participants provided informed consent and were able to ask questions to about the study to the interviewer. Additionally, participants were asked to provide confirmation of HIV status through lab results, medication bottle, or doctor's note. Upon completion of the interview, participants were compensated $40 for their time. The interview guide consisted of questions on personal experiences with HIV, sexual orientation, social networks, transgender identity, aging, substance use, mental health, advanced care planning, and resilience. Each interview took approximately 45–90 minutes to complete. All study activities were approved by the Institutional Review Board at Rutgers, The State University of New Jersey.

4.2 *Data Analysis*

All interviews were audio-recorded and stored on a secure database. Trained research staff (i.e., interns, research assistants, and doctoral students) transcribed and cross-checked all 40 interviews for accuracy. Participant names and identifying information were deleted during transcribing to maintain anonymity. The research team used a multi-step approach to identify and analyze prominent themes from the transcripts. This approach included open coding, application of codes to transcripts and further review of transcripts and codes to identify patterns and themes. Upon completion of coding, quotations were extracted and organized into larger themes based on the patterns discovered during the analysis. With the exception of some minor edits to improve overall clarity and understanding, all quotations are provided verbatim. Qualitative data were coded and organized using Microsoft Excel and Word, and quantitative data on sample characteristics were analyzed using SPSS v28.

5 Results

5.1 *Sociodemographic Characteristics*

The age range of n = 40 participants was 51–69 years old with the mean age being 57.8 years old. The sex divide was relatively split with 55% (n = 22) identifying as male and 45% (n = 18) identifying as female. We do not have any information on the intersex characteristics of the participants. The study overwhelmingly recruited Black individuals (n = 36, 90%) with the remaining participants identifying as white (n = 3, 7.5%) or another race (n = 1, 2.5%).

5.2 *Qualitative Findings: What Is Resilience?*

While the goals of the interviews were multifaceted, one of the main themes we were interested in exploring was the meaning of resilience in the context of being an older adult living with HIV/AIDS. More specifically, we asked each participant, 'in your opinion, what is resilience?,' and we often followed it up with the prompt, 'what does resilience mean to you as a person living with HIV/AIDS? After reviewing the transcripts, three main sub-themes under the resilience domain emerged: (1) health and sobriety; (2) spirituality; and (3) positivity, thriving, and living in the moment.

5.2.1 Theme 1: Health and Sobriety

Given that many of the questions asked during the interview pertained to overall physical and mental health outcomes, it is not surprising that many participants rooted their definitions of resilience in overall health and well-being.

Throughout most of the responses, participants mentioned specific aspects of HIV-related health including their favorable lab results including their CD4 counts and viral load. One participant noted, "My resilience for being diagnosed is to believe that I could still live with this virus...I bounce back—I bounced back from two T-cells to now 100. And if you do the footwork, you'll get results" (Black woman, age 58). Similarly, another participant described the need to improve their HIV-related vitals:

> The ability to come back from a very terrible situation and me being in the situation that I'm in now. Like I was saying I was a mess, I was HIV positive, I had sepsis, I has no T-cells in my body, viral loads 750,000. You know and I was wondering, and the doctor was wondering, 'why am I still walking on this earth?' And so after that I knew I had to decrease this viral load, I knew I had to bring the viral load down, so I would take my medicine every day. (Black man, age 53)

In many of the interviews, participants shared insight around their history of substance use and the myriad steps they've taken to reduce and/or even quit using substances all together. In particular, one participant explained how sobriety was related to their view of resilience:

> It means that I must maintain my sobriety. It means that I must continue to go to groups to learn about new treatments and so forth and so on, and also to give back—to people who just are comin' into the roles, comin' into like a-any meeting, or just comin' into a study group for HIV and AIDS. I must be there to help impact them, you know what I'm sayin', to share my, you know, experiences. (Black man, age 61)

The above example also highlights the importance of social support, community groups, and general mentorship as meaningful ways to maintain overall health and well-being while living with HIV/AIDS.

5.2.2 Theme 2: Spirituality

The second theme that heavily emerged throughout many of the interviews revolves around spirituality, and more specifically being grateful for the role that God and/or another higher power has played in keeping them alive and thriving in the face of adversity. One participant discussed how they often do not think about HIV very often and we found this to be true in several of the interviews:

> I-I just try to stay positive. I-I can't, I can't say it no more, I stay positive. I-I pray every day and that for me works ahh that works for me that-that's my start to just pray and-and thank God, I-I thank him for my life, I-I really don't even think about HIV, you know I-I don't know how other people deal with it but for me, I don't wake up even claiming I have HIV. I just don't, I umm I really just stay positive…I've always been that kinda person…you know there for other people because you know I have my family, I have people who are there for me so I just, I just live my life I-I-I mean I do what makes me…I really honestly don't wake up thinking about HIV. (Black woman, age 53)

Another participant explained that the strength from their relationship with God caused them to bounce back and 'rise like a Phoenix from the ashes' despite facing many other life challenges in addition to living with HIV/AIDS:

> To bounce back. To rise from the ashes like the Phoenix…Yes, and I have risen from the ashes…I mean I'm at a place right now, especially after losing my mother and sister, it would not take much for me to go left. I'm holding on to God's unchanging hand. I'm holding on to what strength I have left because I have to. Because if I don't, I'm-I'm-I'm gonna lose it…so, I'm staying strong, staying in my truth, as the kids would say I'm staying in my truth I'm being um, I'm bouncing back, you know the best way to describe it is like the phoenix rising from the ashes…. (Black man, age 64)

Other participants elucidated that resilience was not only related to their relationship with God, but also with family and other loved ones surrounding them. Without the strength of those relationships, they may not be in the same position with regard to health, security, and overall well-being.

> It's to bounce back cause um I had I think I had pneumonia like 5 or 6 times, but God always brought me back…I ate like I was supposed to, I got the right doctor…and I just-I just give all my glory to God um he had to do it. Um I definitely bounced back quite back a few times…I adopted a son from a month old, he was um my Godson and…he is 22 now and… that's my pride and joy cause I had somebody that loved me for me unconditionally…I d-definitely bounced back so when I got him I felt an even stronger will to live cause I had him to look after you know so that's my bounce back moment was him, my resilience, it was him. I gave it all

> to you know my praise to God for bringing him into my life, uhm and I needed that. (Black man, age 57)

Similar sentiments were echoed by another participant who also added that they overcame past hardships including housing and food instability but that relationships with family and God have helped them turn a corner:

> Man, I struggle. Now I'm on top of my—I'm on top of my-my-my well-being. I got God in my life again, I got mama that love me, I got a wife that love me, you know what I mean? That comes with—uh I had the—eh—going through some stuff man, you know to know that somebody care for me. You know what I mean? I had to lay out in-in the streets out there…I was ashamed man I used to leave down here and go around trying to look for something to eat. Today, I don't have to do that, man. Today, I can go in my ice box and get something to eat. You know um, no man would feel good doing that kind of stuff, man. (Black man, age 69)

5.2.3 Theme 3: Positivity, Thriving, and Living in the Moment

The final theme to emerge around resilience and aging with HIV/AIDS is multifaceted and yet, also interconnected. Many participants explained that resilience is a positive mindset that can help navigate everyday life experiences. One participant used a series of one-word positive affirmations to explain their thoughts about resilience:

> P: Positive. Good things. Growth. Maturity. Respect…and to treat others how you would want to be treated.
>
> I: And why did you choose those words and phrases?
>
> P: I choose those words and those phrases because I use that in my everyday life. In my everyday life. And I try to give, I try to-to be an example of that and to give that fact because as people give it to me it's not enough for me to just keep it and be selfish with it and don't share it back. (Black man, age 59)

Similarly, another participant rationalized resilience as being able to turn something that is often considered to be negative (e.g., living with HIV/AIDS) into a positive situation, while helping others in the process:

> Resilience means to me means that I have overcome a negative, a real bad negative attitude towards everything and everybody. When I found out I was [HIV-]positive, I realized that I couldn't live like that anymore. I couldn't um keep walking around with that attitude, wanting to fight. Cussing and carrying on, it was just not me. So, I turned that negative into a positive and now I want to help people. You know back then I didn't want to be bothered by nobody, I didn't want to help nobody. I didn't want to talk to nobody but now it's like I can talk about it about it today. I can help people today with it. (Black woman, age 55)

Other participants echoed sentiments about bouncing back from adverse situations and are now not just surviving but rather thriving while overcoming past obstacles and turning them into opportunities to create a better life for themselves:

> Resilience is who I am…I came from homelessness to uhh, to living a fairly decent normal life. I mean I have a Master's degree in science. I went back to school got my undergrad and my graduate degree from homelessness and crack addiction. I was living in a tent on the lower East side of Manhattan, you know in the middle of the winter with a hibachi keeping me warm…[now] I have a four-bedroom house with a swimming pool in the back and two BMWs and you know, I think I am the definition of resilience. (Black man, age 64)

As another participant explained, resilience can also mean not giving up, despite different trials and tribulations.

> Resilience means for me, as I say is never giving up! I've never given up on life, I've never given up on my ability to create, my worth, my talent, which I still fight for, with people still questioning and challenging but I know what I know, I know, from experience, from education, and my intuitive sense that secures my confidence and motivation and to always feel like I'm on top of my game, now to be able to articulate the English language proudly and correctly, share my thoughts and knowledge and stuff. That secures my confidence and my drive and my resilience, and uh, um, yeah…the first year of college I was on the dean's list, I wanted it so bad! (Black man, age 58)

Finally, several participants discussed resilience as living in the moment and enjoying life to its fullest, especially since many did not plan on living into older age. For some, this involves planning future vacations or spontaneous outings on a Saturday afternoon:

> Keep pushing. Go after what I-what I want. Um, don't settle for less. There are things out there that I want to do. Um, the other thing is I always wanted to go to Hawaii, so, go ahead and do. Um, my husband and I always travel. We-We'll just jump up and say, "okay let's do that," you know. We push off each other you know. Um, like last Saturday, he was like oh I'm getting off, what you wanna do? He-I'm like I just want to relax. He was like 'it's nice out-it was beautiful outside'...So, we jump up and we go to Philly...You know, that's honest...just-just do it. (Black woman, age 60)

Likewise, another participant emphasized that living with HIV is not the death sentence that it was once considered by simply stating, "resilience for me is determination um and the ability to ya know realize that it doesn't have to be the end..." (Black woman, age 54).

6 Discussion and Implications

These findings presented here focus on many different aspects of how resilience is operationalized by older adults aging with HIV/AIDS. Virtually all participants had some sort of definition as to what resilience meant to them and many were able to connect their thoughts back to overcoming the challenges association with HIV and focusing on how they have not only survived but also thrived in the face of adversity. As such, there are several things about that researchers, providers, and practitioners, should consider when thinking about resilience in the context of aging with HIV.

6.1 *Resilience as an Underutilized Approach*

The sentiments shared in these interviews underscore the need to utilize resilience as a tool among aging populations, especially those living with HIV/AIDS. For example, studies of older adults have found that strong social ties are associated with increased levels of resilience (Netuveli et al., 2008; Wells, 2012). As noted by a couple of participants, social and familial support played a key role in operationalizing what resilience meant to them. An intervention or program utilizing social support, or a group-based activity could help activate untapped resources or harness existing processes to increase resilience among older PLWHA. This also speaks to care that is not just biological but is more biopsychosocial in its approach.

Resilience can also be utilized as a tool to both normalize living with HIV/AIDS. As demonstrated in other studies (Krause, 2020), HIV-related resilience acted as a mediator between the impact of HIV-related stigma and mental health outcomes. A recent set of meta-analyses found significant associations between HIV-related stigma and fewer social support resources and higher rates of depression (Rueda et al., 2016). Using resilience as a way to lessen the impact of HIV-related stigma could be a necessary point of intervention. Furthermore, a resilience-based approach enables us to examine health more holistically with regard to a biopsychosocial approach.

6.2 *Public Health: Sifting from a Deficits-Based to a Strengths-Based Approach*

For decades, public health practitioners and researchers have predominantly studied health conditions and outcomes from a deficits-based perspective (Morgan & Ziglio, 2007). In general, there is a wide-ranging understanding and consensus around the social conditions and factors—apart from medical ones—that drive health across settings and populations (Braveman & Gottlieb, 2014). From poverty to racism, and from educational inequities to homophobia, these structural barriers have often driven public health theory, practice, and policy. However, while these foci are vitally important and necessary, deficit models tend to define individuals and communities negatively while often disregarding what works well and is positive within a particular population (Morgan & Ziglio, 2007).

The majority of research on PLWHA, and especially gay, bisexual and other MSM who are aging and members of the AIDS Generation (i.e., those who came of age in the 1980s at the height of the HIV/AIDS epidemic) (Halkitis, 2013) has focused extensively on risk. Other research has concentrated on complications and the negative ramifications of being diagnosed and/or living with HIV/AIDS (i.e., what is wrong with living with HIV/AIDS and not what the positive aspects may be). Those who are part of the AIDS Generation are entering uncharted territory—they are living far longer than many of them expected considering how many of them lost their colleagues, friends, partners, and lovers from AIDS-related complications prior to the development and implementation of ART. Research confirming the myriad challenges and difficulties of living with HIV/AIDS is not needed because they know far too well—these individuals have lived it for the last three decades in one way or another. The resilience this community exhibits both individually and collectively is unmatched to any other impacted by an epidemic in modern history. Similar sentiments were echoed by several participants, especially when discussing how important social support and groups were to overcoming issues such as substance use and economic instability. As such, it is critically important for public health researchers and practitioners to focus on and refine the resilience paradigm within older PLWHA so that it can serve as a blueprint for a healthier and more meaningful journey of aging.

6.3 *Healthcare for Older PLWHA*

As PLWHA age, their biopsychosocial healthcare challenges will become more complex (Miller et al., 2019; Mugavero et al., 2009). Mugavero and colleagues (2009) outline a socioecological perspective of multilevel factors that influence the processes of engagement in care. In this model, individual factors such as mental health, comorbidities, and resiliency are layered with relationships, community (including the healthcare system) and policies (i.e., Ryan White CARE Act, Affordable Care Act, and other quality measures/indicators). Navigating the structural and interpersonal dynamics can be challenging for anyone, but PLWHA may face additional psychosocial burdens such as HIV-related stigma that make it more complicated.

In general, the healthcare workforce is not equipped to handle the aging population at-large (Dall et al., 2013; Milani & Lavie, 2015). More specifically, those who work with PLWHA are also overextended and undertrained to manage the aging HIV epidemic (Boccher-Lattimore et al., 2019; Copeland et al., 2017). In other parts of the interviews, participants noted strong relationships with their medical providers, but others had mixed experiences. The majority of respondents to a workforce development survey consisting of HIV experts, clinicians, and leaders indicated that 'HIV and mental health' is the most urgent training need for practitioners working with PLWHA (Boccher-Lattimore et al., 2019). Incorporating resilience and strengths-based perspectives into this training would provide healthcare workers with an important perspective of approaches to holistic care, especially for aging PLWHA.

6.4 *Ending the HIV/AIDS Epidemic*

As noted previously, the United States federal government initiated a nationwide 'Ending the HIV Epidemic (EtE)' initiative in 2019 (HIV.gov, 2022). In order to truly end the epidemic, plans must support PLWHA (Adams & Flood, 2019) by addressing mental health and substance use (Remien et al., 2019) especially because these health-related challenges may impact adherence to ART (Neigh et al., 2016; Samuels et al., 2011). Disruption to antiretroviral treatment will significantly impact the final stage of the HIV continuum of care and will make widespread viral suppression extremely difficult to achieve, especially by 2030. The challenge with many of the current EtE plans is that they mainly focus on the virus itself and not the person living with the virus. With that, the findings from these interviews demonstrate the need to support PLWHA as people and not as incubators of a virus.

6.5 *Bridging the Gap: The Health of Populations and Individuals*

With the relatively recent movement towards translational research that focuses on fostering more cohesive relationships between basic scientists and clinical researchers (Rubio et al., 2010), a logical next step is a multidisciplinary approach to research on resilience among older PLWHA. More specifically, public health researchers and practitioners need to work more intentionally with mental health providers and social workers in order to better address the needs of individuals and the population at large. They need to understand that that a person living with HIV/AIDS is not the virus itself. Combining a dynamic public health model that methodically thinks about how each point of intervention informs the next with a psychological approach that focuses on details and depth of underlying causes of problems can be a formidable balance (DeAngelis, 2001). While tending to the needs of individuals is crucial to improving the health of populations, there can also be a synergistic relationship by improving structural and population-based impediments of health that has a direct impact on people. This relationship can be fostered by implementing multi-level resilience interventions and programs that address the interplay among individuals, communities, and the environment at-large.

6.6 *Older PLWHA Are Surviving and Thriving*

One of the most palpable takeaways from these interviews is that people who are aging with HIV/AIDS and living much longer than projected at the onset of the epidemic are not just surviving, but they are thriving. Too often, aging PLWHA have had to overcome immense obstacles throughout their lives in order to live to see another day, make it to another doctor's appointment, and/or ensure financial and housing stability. Collectively, these participants show a relentless spirit to thrive despite the myriad challenges that have often come before them, whether it is a low CD4 count, fractured relationships, or struggles with substance use. They also demonstrate that resilience can be depicted in many forms and is often not a one-size-fits-all approach. It might mean saying yes to a husband's request to take a day trip to Philadelphia or going back to school to get a Bachelor's and Master's degree after living in a tent in Manhattan. It might mean rising from the ashes like the Phoenix or living to be 69 when treatment options were non-existent at time of initial diagnosis. Taken together, resilience can be an incredible tool that helps to support people in the midst of various life challenges, and future research should begin to examine the best mechanisms for interventions and programs to ensure longevity for all PLWHA.

7 Conclusions

The findings from these interviews can help us better understand how resilience is operationalized among older adults living with HIV/AIDS. Resilience-focused interventions, programs, and policies need to be developed for older adults living with HIV/AIDS and may be improved by targeting the mental health and substance use challenges identified in these interviews by tapping into opportunities for increased social and community support. Moreover, bringing public health researchers and practitioners together with mental health providers and clinicians will help bridge the gap between disciplines and approaches to care. Furthermore, this re-alignment will help shift conversations within the public health field towards a strengths-based approach instead of focusing predominantly on deficits. Finally, it is important to acknowledge that older PLWHA are not merely surviving. Rather, many are increasingly thriving as they age and continue to make sense of how living with HIV/AIDS has shaped their lives.

Acknowledgements

I would like to thank Dr. Perry N. Halkitis for his constant guidance and support as I have navigated this research space for the last six years. Additionally, I would like to acknowledge all of the participants who agreed to be part of this study for sharing their invaluable insights and perspectives with myself and other members of the team at the Center for Health, Identity, Behavior and Prevention Studies (CHIBPS).

References

Adams, M., & Flood, A. (2019). Ending the HIV epidemic requires supporting those already living with HIV. *Morning Consult*. https://morningconsult.com/opinions/ending-hiv-epidemic-requires-supporting-those-already-living-with-hiv/

Azar, A. (2019, March 20). *Ending the HIV epidemic: A plan for America*. https://www.hhs.gov/blog/2019/02/05/ending-the-hiv-epidemic-a-plan-for-america.html

Bhatia, M., & Munjal, S. (2014). Prevalence of depression in people living with HIV/AIDS undergoing ART and factors associated with it. *Journal of Clinical and Diagnostic Research*, *8*(10), WC01–04. https://doi.org/10.7860/jcdr/2014/7725.4927

Bird, S. T., Bogart, L. M., & Delahanty, D. L. (2004). Health-related correlates of perceived discrimination in HIV care. *AIDS Patient Care and STDs*, *18*(1), 19–26. https://www.liebertpub.com/doi/abs/10.1089/108729104322740884

Blanco, J. R., Jarrín, I., Vallejo, M., Berenguer, J., Solera, C., Rubio, R., Pulido, F., Asensi, V., del Amo, J., Moreno, & CoRis, S. (2012). Definition of advanced age in HIV infection: Looking for an age cut-off. *AIDS Research and Human Retroviruses*, *28*(9), 1000–1006. https://www.ncbi.nlm.nih.gov/pmc/articles/PMC3423793/pdf/aid.2011.0377.pdf

Boccher-Lattimore, D., Millery, M., McKinnon, K., Li, M., & Cournos, F. (2019). Workforce development needs in HIV care: A response to mental health and HIV/AIDS: the need for an integrated response. *Aids*, *33*(13), 2109–2110.

Brandt, C., Zvolensky, M. J., Woods, S. P., Gonzalez, A., Safren, S. A., & O'Cleirigh, C. M. (2017). Anxiety symptoms and disorders among adults living with HIV and AIDS: A critical review and integrative synthesis of the empirical literature. *Clinical Psychology Review*, *51*, 164–184. https://doi.org/10.1016/j.cpr.2016.11.005

Braveman, P., & Gottlieb, L. (2014). The social determinants of health: It's time to consider the causes of the causes. *Public Health Reports*, *129* (Suppl 2), 19–31. https://doi.org/10.1177/00333549141291s206

Buttram, M. E. (2015). The social environmental elements of resilience among vulnerable African American/Black men who have sex with men. *Journal of Human Behavior in the Social Environment*, *25*(8), 923–933. https://doi.org/10.1080/10911359.2015.1040908

Centers for Disease Control and Prevention. (2019). *HIV Among people aged 50 and over.* The Centers for Disease Control and Prevention. Retrieved March 21, 2021, from http://www.cdc.gov/hiv/group/age/olderamericans/index.html

Centers for Disease Control and Prevention. (2022). *HIV Surveillance Report, 2020.* https://www.cdc.gov/hiv/library/reports/hiv-surveillance.html.

Clifford, D. B., & Ances, B. M. (2013). HIV-associated neurocognitive disorder. *The Lancet Infectious Diseases*, *13*(11), 976–986. https://doi.org/10.1016/s1473-3099(13)70269-x

Comas-Diaz, L., Luthar, S. S., Maddi, S. R., O'Neill, H. K., Saakvitne, K. W., & Tedeschi, R. G. (2004). *The road to resilience.* American Psychological Association.

Copeland, R. M., Wilson, P., Betancourt, G., Garcia, D., Penner, M., Abravanel, R., Wong, E. Y., & Parisi, L. D. (2017). Disparities in HIV knowledge and attitudes toward biomedical interventions among the non-medical HIV workforce in the United States. *AIDS Care*, *29*(12), 1576–1584.

Dall, T. M., Gallo, P. D., Chakrabarti, R., West, T., Semilla, A. P., & Storm, M. V. (2013). An aging population and growing disease burden will require alarge and specialized health care workforce by 2025. *Health Affairs*, *32*(11), 2013–2020.

DeAngelis, T. (2001). *A successful marriage of psychology and public health.* American Psychological Association. https://www.apa.org/monitor/mar01/publichealth

De Santis, J. P., Florom-Smith, A., Vermeesch, A., Barroso, S., & DeLeon, D. A. (2013). Motivation, management, and mastery: A theory of resilience in the context of HIV infection. *Journal of the American Psychiatric Nurses Association, 19*(1), 36–46. https://doi.org/10.1177/1078390312474096

Emlet, C. A. (2006). "You're awfully old to have this disease": Experiences of stigma and ageism in adults 50 years and older living with HIV/AIDS. *The Gerontologist, 46*(6), 781–790.

Emlet, C. A., Tozay, S., & Raveis, V. (2011). "I'm not going to die from the AIDS": Resilience in aging with HIV disease. *Gerontologist, 51*(1), 101–111. https://doi.org/10.1093/geront/gnq060

Ford, C. L., Daniel, M., Earp, J. A., Kaufman, J. S., Golin, C. E., & Miller, W. C. (2009). Perceived everyday racism, residential segregation, and HIV testing among patients at a sexually transmitted disease clinic. *American Journal of Public Health, 99*(Suppl 1), S137–143.

Garcia-Dia, M. J., DiNapoli, J. M., Garcia-Ona, L., Jakubowski, R., & O'Flaherty, D. (2013). Concept analysis: Resilience. *Archives of Psychiatric Nursing, 27*(6), 264–270. https://doi.org/10.1016/j.apnu.2013.07.003

Goldstein, S., & Brooks, R. B. (2013). Why study resilience? In S. Goldstein & R. B. Brooks (Eds.), *Handbook of resilience in children* (pp. 3–14). Springer.

Gonzalez, J. S., Batchelder, A. W., Psaros, C., & Safren, S. A. (2011). Depression and HIV/AIDS treatment nonadherence: A review and meta-analysis. *JAIDS Journal of Acquired Immune Deficiency Syndromes, 58*(2), 181–187. https://doi.org/10.1097/QAI.0b013e31822d490a

Gooding, P. A., Hurst, A., Johnson, J., & Tarrier, N. (2012). Psychological resilience in young and older adults. *International Journal of Geriatric Psychiatry, 27*(3), 262–270. https://doi.org/10.1002/gps.2712

Grov, C., Golub, S. A., Parsons, J. T., Brennan, M., & Karpiak, S. E. (2010). Loneliness and HIV-related stigma explain depression among older HIV-positive adults. *AIDS Care, 22*(5), 630–639. https://doi.org/10.1080/09540120903280901

Guaraldi, G., Zona, S., Brothers, T. D., Carli, F., Stentarelli, C., Dolci, G., Santoro, A., Beghetto, B., Menozzi, M., & Mussini, C. (2015). Aging with HIV vs. HIV seroconversion at older age: A diverse population with distinct comorbidity profiles. *PLoS One, 10*(4), e0118531. https://www.ncbi.nlm.nih.gov/pmc/articles/PMC4395353/pdf/pone.0118531.pdf

Halkitis, P. N. (2013). *The AIDS generation: Stories of survival and resilience.* Oxford University Press.

Halkitis, P. N., Krause, K. D., & Vieira, D. L. (2017). Mental health, psychosocial challenges and resilience in older adults living with HIV. In M. Brennan-Ing & R. F. DeMarco (Eds.), *HIV and aging* (pp. 187–203). Karger. https://doi.org/10.1159/000448564

Hassani, P., Izadi-Avanji, F. S., Rakhshan, M., & Majd, H. A. (2017). A phenomenological study on resilience of the elderly suffering from chronic disease: A qualitative study. *Psychology Research and Behavior Management*, *10*, 59–67. https://doi.org/10.2147/prbm.S121336

Herek, G. M., Gillis, J. R., & Cogan, J. C. (2009). Internalized stigma among sexual minority adults: Insights from a social psychological perspective. *Journal of Counseling Psychology*, *56*(1), 32–43. https://doi.org/10.1037/a0014672

Herrick, A. L., Lim, S. H., Wei, C., Smith, H., Guadamuz, T., Friedman, M. S., & Stall, R. (2011). Resilience as an untapped resource in behavioral intervention design for gay men. *AIDS and Behaviour*, *15*(Suppl 1), S25–S29. https://doi.org/10.1007/s10461-011-9895-0

Hildon, Z., Montgomery, S. M., Blane, D., Wiggins, R. D., & Netuveli, G. (2010). Examining resilience of quality of life in the face of health-related and psychosocial adversity at older ages: What is "right" about the way we age? *Gerontologist*, *50*(1), 36–47. https://doi.org/10.1093/geront/gnp067

HIV.gov. (2022). *U.S. statistics*. U.S. Department of Health & Human Services. Retrieved August 31, 2021, from https://www.hiv.gov/federal-response/ending-the-hiv-epidemic/overview

Hussen, S. A., Tsegaye, M., Argaw, M. G., Andes, K., Gilliard, D., & del Rio, C. (2014). Spirituality, social capital and service: Factors promoting resilience among Expert Patients living with HIV in Ethiopia. *Global Public Health*, *9*(3), 286–298. https://doi.org/10.1080/17441692.2014.880501

Jang, H., Anderson, P. G., & Mentes, J. C. (2011). Aging and living with HIV/AIDS. *Journal of Gerontological Nursing*, *37*(12), 4–7. https://doi.org/10.3928/00989134-20111104-02

Jeste, D. V., Savla, G. N., Thompson, W. K., Vahia, I. V., Glorioso, D. K., Martin, A. S., Palmer, B. W., Rock, D., Golshan, S., Kraemer, H. C., & Depp, C. A. (2013). Association between older age and more successful aging: critical role of resilience and depression. *The American Journal of Psychiatry*, *170*(2), 188–196. https://doi.org/10.1176/appi.ajp.2012.12030386

Justice, A. C., & Tate, J. P. (2019). Ageing with and without HIV: Will advanced age bring equity or greater disparity? *Journal of the International AIDS Society*, *22*(9), e25400. https://doi.org/10.1002/jia2.25400

Krause, K. D. (2020). *Resilience as a buffer against negative health sequelae in older gay men living with HIV/AIDS: Implications for research and practice*. Rutgers School of Graduate Studies.

Leng, S. X., & Margolick, J. B. (2015). Understanding frailty, aging, and inflammation in HIV infection. *Current HIV/AIDS Reports*, *12*(1), 25–32. https://doi.org/10.1007/s11904-014-0247-3

Levin, J. (2012). *Comorbidty and ageing with HIV: A prospective comparitive cohort study* [Paper]. XIX International AIDS Conference, Washington, DC. http://www.natap.org/2012/IAS/IAS_55.htm

Luthar, S. S., & Cicchetti, D. (2000). The construct of resilience: Implications for interventions and social policies. *Development and Psychopathology, 12*(4), 857–885.

MacLeod, S., Musich, S., Hawkins, K., Alsgaard, K., & Wicker, E. R. (2016). The impact of resilience among older adults. *Geriatric Nursing, 37*(4), 266–272. https://doi.org/10.1016/j.gerinurse.2016.02.014

Mahale, P., Engels, E. A., Coghill, A. E., Kahn, A. R., & Shiels, M. S. (2018). Cancer risk in older persons living with human immunodeficiency virus infection in the United States. *Clinical Infectious Diseases, 67*(1), 50–57. https://doi.org/10.1093/cid/ciy012

Marion, M. (1996). Living in an era of multiple loss and trauma: Understanding global loss in the gay community. In C. J. Alexander (Ed.), *Gay and lesbian mental health: A sourcebook for practitioners* (pp. 61–93). Routledge.

Masten, A. S., & Wright, M. O. (2010). Resilience over the lifespan: Developmental perspectives on resistance, recovery, and transformation. In J. W. Reich, A. J. Zautra, & J. S. Hall (Eds.), *Handbook of adult resilience* (pp. 213–237). The Guilford Press.

Masten, J., & Schmidtberger, J. (2011). *Aging with HIV: A gay man's guide.* Oxford University Press.

Milani, R. V., & Lavie, C. J. (2015). Health care 2020: Reengineering health care delivery to combat chronic disease. *The American Journal of Medicine, 128*(4), 337–343.

Miller, T. R., Halkitis, P. N., & Durvasula, R. (2019). A biopsychosocial approach to managing HIV-related pain and associated substance abuse in older adults: a review. *Ageing International, 44*(1), 74–116.

Morgan, A., & Ziglio, E. (2007). Revitalising the evidence base for public health: An assets model. *Promototion and Education, 14*(Suppl. 2), 17–22. https://doi.org/10.1177/10253823070140020701x

Mugavero, M. J., Lin, H.-Y., Willig, J. H., Westfall, A. O., Ulett, K. B., Routman, J. S., Abroms, S., Raper, J. L., Saag, M. S., & Allison, J. J. (2009). Missed visits and mortality among patients establishing initial outpatient HIV treatment. *Clinical Infectious Diseases, 48*(2), 248–256.

Neigh, G. N., Rhodes, S. T., Valdez, A., & Jovanovic, T. (2016). PTSD co-morbid with HIV: Separate but equal, or two parts of a whole? *Neurobiology of Diseases, 92*(Pt B), 116–123. https://doi.org/10.1016/j.nbd.2015.11.012

Netuveli, G., & Blane, D. (2008). Quality of life in older ages. *British Medical Bulletin, 85*(1), 113–126.

Netuveli, G., Wiggins, R. D., Montgomery, S. M., Hildon, Z., & Blane, D. (2008). Mental health and resilience at older ages: Bouncing back after adversity in the British Household Panel Survey. *Journal of Epidemiology and Community Health, 62*(11), 987–991. https://doi.org/10.1136/jech.2007.069138

Orton, L., Griffiths, J., Green, M., & Waterman, H. (2012). Resilience among asylum seekers living with HIV. *BMC Public Health, 12*, 926. https://doi.org/10.1186/1471-2458-12-926

Owen, G., & Catalan, J. (2012). 'We never expected this to happen': narratives of ageing with HIV among gay men living in London, UK. *Culture, Health & Sexuality*, *14*(1), 59–72. https://doi.org/10.1080/13691058.2011.621449

Remien, R. H., & Rabkin, J. G. (2001). Psychological aspects of living with HIV disease: A primary care perspective. *The Western Journal of Medicine*, *175*(5), 332–335. https://www.ncbi.nlm.nih.gov/pmc/articles/PMC1071613/pdf/wjm17500332.pdf

Remien, R. H., Stirratt, M. J., Nguyen, N., Robbins, R. N., Pala, A. N., & Mellins, C. A. (2019). Mental health and HIV/AIDS: The need for an integrated response. *Aids*, *33*(9), 1411.

Resnick, B. A. (2018). The relationship between resilience and motivation. In B. Resnick, L. Gwyther, & R. K. (Eds.), *Resilience in aging: Concepts, research, and outcomes* (pp. 199–215). Springer.

Resnick, B. A., & Inguito, P. L. (2011). The resilience scale: Psychometric properties and clinical applicability in older adults. *Archives of Psychiatric Nursing*, *25*(1), 11–20. https://doi.org/10.1016/j.apnu.2010.05.001

Riedel, D. J., Tang, L. S., & Rositch, A. F. (2015). The role of viral co-infection in HIV-associated non-AIDS-related cancers. *Current HIV/AIDS Reports*, *12*(3), 362–372. https://doi.org/10.1007/s11904-015-0276-6

Robinson, W. A., Petty, M. S., Patton, C., & Kang, H. (2008). Aging with HIV: Historical and intra-community differences in experience of aging with HIV. *Journal of Gay & Lesbian Social Services*, *20*(1–2), 111–128.

Rubio, D. M., Schoenbaum, E. E., Lee, L. S., Schteingart, D. E., Marantz, P. R., Anderson, K. E., Platt, L. D., Baez, A., & Esposito, K. (2010). Defining translational research: Implications for training. *Academic Medicine*, *85*(3), 470–475. https://doi.org/10.1097/ACM.0b013e3181ccd618

Rueda, S., Mitra, S., Chen, S., Gogolishvili, D., Globerman, J., Chambers, L., Wilson, M., Logie, C. H., Shi, Q., & Morassaei, S. (2016). Examining the associations between HIV-related stigma and health outcomes in people living with HIV/AIDS: A series of meta-analyses. *BMJ open*, *6*(7), e011453.

Samuels, E., Khalife, S., Alfonso, C. A., Alvarez, R., & Cohen, M. A. (2011). Early childhood trauma, posttraumatic stress disorder, and non-adherence in persons with AIDS: A psychodynamic perspective. *The Journal of the American Academy of Psychoanalys and Dynamic Psychiatry*, *39*(4), 633–650. https://doi.org/10.1521/jaap.2011.39.4.633

Sayles, J. N., Ryan, G. W., Silver, J. S., Sarkisian, C. A., & Cunningham, W. E. (2007). Experiences of social stigma and implications for healthcare among a diverse population of HIV positive adults. *Journal of Urban Health*, *84*(6), 814–828. https://www.ncbi.nlm.nih.gov/pmc/articles/PMC2232034/pdf/11524_2007_Article_9220.pdf

Shen, K., & Zeng, Y. (2011). The association between resilience and survival among Chinese elderly. In B. Resnick, L. P. Gwyther, & K. A. Roberto (Eds.), *Resilience in aging* (pp. 217–229). Springer.

Siegel, K., Raveis, V. H., & Karus, D. (1998). Perceived advantages and disadvantages of age among older HIV-infected adults. *Research on Aging*, *20*(6), 686–711.

Simone, M. J., & Appelbaum, J. (2008). HIV in older adults. *Geriatrics*, *63*(12), 6–12.

Smith, J. L., & Hollinger-Smith, L. (2015). Savoring, resilience, and psychological well-being in older adults. *Aging & Mental Health*, *19*(3), 192–200.

Tkatch, R., Musich, S., MacLeod, S., Kraemer, S., Hawkins, K., Wicker, E. R., & Armstrong, D. G. (2017). A qualitative study to examine older adults' perceptions of health: Keys to aging successfully. *Geriatric Nursing*, *38*(6), 485–490.

UNAIDS. (2022). *Fact sheet 2022: Global HIV statistics*. https://www.unaids.org/sites/default/files/media_asset/UNAIDS_FactSheet_en.pdf

Wallach, I. (2011). "I am happy for having the age that I have": The resilience of gay aged men living with HIV in Quebec. *Canadian Journal of Community Mental Health*, *30*(2), 157–171.

Wells, M. (2012). Resilience in older adults living in rural, suburban, and urban areas. *Online Journal of Rural Nursing and Health Care*, *10*(2), 45–54.

Youmans, E., Tripathi, A., Gibson, J. J., Stephens, T., & Duffus, W. A. (2011). Demographic characteristics and behavioral risk factors of HIV infection and association with survival among individuals 50 years or older. *Southern Medical Journal*, *104*(10), 669–675. https://doi.org/10.1097/SMJ.0b013e31822dd3d8

Zicari, S., Sessa, L., Cotugno, N., Ruggiero, A., Morrocchi, E., Concato, C., Rocca, S., Zangari, P., Manno, E. C., & Palma, P. (2019). Immune activation, inflammation, and non-AIDS co-morbidities in HIV-infected patients under long-term ART. *Viruses*, *11*(3). https://doi.org/10.3390/v11030200

CHAPTER 6

Embracing and Authentic Feminine Self

Angela Hunt (with Audria LB)

My name is Angela ZanieYa Hunt, and this is my story.

I was born on June 4th, 1979, to my mother Gladys Smith and my father, who is still unknown to me. I was the second child, named Frederick Antonio Smith, after Frederick Douglass. My grandmother named me Miss Irene Graham. My story, like so many others, started off as what most of us would call "normal." We knew that they loved, cared for, and nurtured us. For most of my life growing up, I was raised by my auntie and my sister. We didn't have the best life, but it was a safe one; until one day, when my sister and I were playing by my grandmother's window. My grandmother had worked a few days in a row with no sleep, and so she woke up very upset and angry. My mother had come back to stay with us at this time. She didn't know what to do, so the first thing she did was to grab a cord from the back of the TV and beat us for waking our grandmother. My sister ran away and ended up at one of our teachers' houses around the corner. Police and Child Protective Services were called, and we were soon placed into foster care.

After being placed in foster care, our lives began to change. At times, it was just me and my sister, and they initially tried to place us with family that would take us both. So we journeyed back and forth between family relatives and foster care homes. They did everything they could to keep us together, and for the most part, we did. I always depended on my sister. I did everything she did, played with what she played with, and soon I began to realize that I was not like other boys. I loved playing with dolls, I loved playing house, I loved playing store clerk. We used to get the big JCPenney catalogs when I was younger, and we would act like sales reps on the phone selling items. We would build this little big top tent in our rooms, and just enjoy ourselves playing sales clerk.

Our foster mother at the time became very ill, and so we went back into the foster care system. This time, we lucked out and ended up going to stay at my sister's father's house with his family, because we stayed in the same city at the time. We stayed together for a few more years. I was so happy that I had a sister and brother who were both older than me. But while I was happy, it turned out that no one else was. I was told that it had become too expensive to take care of three teenagers, and that changes had to be made. Well, that change was to

 | DOI:10.1163/9789004708136_007

send me back to foster care. My life changed forever, and from this day forward I always felt abandoned.

I could not help but feel that everyone in my life wanted nothing to do with me. I was placed in and then moved from one house to another for several years, until one of my foster mothers told me I needed to straighten up, because no one's gonna take care of a child who burns down houses. This was news to me! I had no idea what she was talking about or what she meant. So, in one of my therapy sessions, the therapist pulled up my file and said yes, that I was labeled as an arsonist. We talked about it and she tried to help me, but I quickly shut down. I never forgot, though. I've always thought about it, but I never brought it up because I didn't want anyone to dislike me.

I continued to be passed along from house to house. There was one foster family that was willing to take care of me, but at this point I had a reputation for taking my anger out on others. Now not only had I been labeled an arsonist, but I was also labeled a troubled child at school. I got caught up in a lot of fights, most of them to defend people who I had called friends, but nevertheless I was still caught in the middle of them. They felt that I had become unmanageable and that I needed better resources, so they sent me to A. Quinn Jones, a school for children with learning disabilities and behavioral problems. I met a teacher there who inspired me to change, no matter what. And to top it all off, I got placed in a foster home with a family who truly showed love and support. I remember sitting down and going over my records, and them taking my records and locking them up in a file, saying they no longer exist. Then they told me to trust God and trust the process, to remember to always let go of all hate and pain, and to love my family no matter what.

Throughout my middle and high school years, I was considered a bad child. I went to a behavior school where I broke my arm pulling back from a teacher to defend a friend. I made so many mistakes, but what most people did not realize is that I was doing it to show people they were loved and supported. Once I developed my group of friends, we became a close friend group who looked out for each other no matter what. We performed in many school activities as a group, and did very well. Eventually, I did well in this program and school setting. Learning disabilities have been a part of my story as well. I learned at a slower pace than most others, and I had to in order to get a clear understanding of what I was reading. When I made it back to my high school, I noticed that I identified more and more with the girls, and got along with them more than anyone else. I felt natural being with my group of friends and my godsister, all of them cisgender girls. I didn't know the word "cisgender" at the time, but I did know that I was one of the girls. We became a family. I did amazing things in school, excelled even with my learning disabilities, and I graduated in the top 25% of my class. Right outta high school, I started working at Boston Market and going to school full time, but that quickly changed when I got a job as a custodian at Shands Hospital in Gainesville, FL. The staff in the pharmacy quarters took notice of me, and made me an offer to join their training course for pharmacy technicians, all paid by Shands. I took on the role, graduated at the top of my class, and was then offered a position as a pharmaceutical technician in the lab. I worked there for about five years. They also trained me in outpatient pharmacy. My knowledge of drugs kept me away from exploring while I was in college, but that time soon ended. This is where my story started to go downhill.

I transferred from my custodian job at Shands Hospital, and began as a pharmaceutical technician trainee. I excelled, but in doing so, I also learned a lot about drugs. I decided at the time that I would not involve myself in illegal or drug activities. At this time, I was also performing three nights a week as a drag queen at the University Club. This, on top of a full-time job and fifteen hours of school per week, started to take a toll on me. Like so many others, I looked for something to help me stay focused, and that something ended up being drugs. They'd keep us awake and alert, but they'd keep us on edge too. I started to fail out of school, and so like any other smart student would, I decided to walk away from my education. I felt like I was on the right track—I was working as a pharmacy technician at Shands Hospital, one of the biggest hospitals in the nation. Soon, they offered me an opportunity to go to school to become a pharmacist, all expenses paid. But I wasn't able to take on this opportunity. Things were going downhill for me with drugs and alcohol, and other problems outside of work were affecting everything around me. My best friend had moved away to Orlando, and six months later I decided to join him. There, I started partying more, to the extent that I began to feel as though life was nothing but a chance to party, club, and enjoy myself. This lifestyle consumed me; I was out of control and getting in trouble with the law. And yet, I felt like that could change, too, that I could party and have fun and make this life work for me. I hit rock bottom, which for me meant realizing that I was a major addict who would do drugs anywhere, in front of anyone, and not care what anyone had to say about it.

To make things worse, a scare I had in 2011 came back to haunt me. Now that I was HIV+, after fighting so hard to accept it the first time I was told that I'd been exposed, I became reckless and careless with my actions, not realizing how much harm it was causing me until it was too late. The lesson I learned was that you don't have to be a slut, freak, or nasty person to contract HIV; all you have to do is not use a condom once with someone who is HIV+, and then you run the risk of becoming HIV+ yourself.

I beat myself up over this, over and over again, feeling as though I had done something terrible. I became more and more involved with drugs, and stopped caring if I came home. My best friend asked me if I would go to rehab if the chance was offered, and I said yes. That morning, he picked me up and took me to rehab for my first stay. I missed everyone, I missed having my own space, and I missed love. I went back to rehab three more times with my wife-to-be, and as of today, I have been clean for 3½ years. It hasn't been easy being trans, HIV+, and living in the streets. It's been a hard struggle, but I stayed connected with my community, who catapulted me into a better space. I am now a health educator with the Hope and Help Center, which has brought me so many wonderful moments in my life, and has empowered me to inspire others. Not only do I see myself as an advocate for my community, I also see myself as a positive role model for those who may have experienced what I've been through. I love and enjoy being a peer support, because it is through them that I find help navigating through my own life. I am now working very hard with my community to provide space and housing opportunities for folks who identify as trans and/or nonbinary and are dealing with homelessness and drug/alcohol addiction, by the end of 2021.

CHAPTER 7

Fathers Who Have Adult Children with Developmental Disabilities Living in Their Home and Their Relationships with Them

A Qualitative Study

Kirsten L. Ostergren Clark

According to a recent Pew report (Parker & Livingston, 2018), fatherhood and the roles fathers play in their children's lives have changed in recent years. A key finding was that fathers are more involved with their children today compared to previous cohorts. Fathers also see parenting as vital to their identity and are spending more time doing child-care and household-related chores (e.g., cleaning and cooking) compared to fifty years ago (Parker & Livingston, 2018). As sociologist Stephen Williams writes, "Fatherhood is increasingly becoming a site of complex structural and personal responsibilities" (2008, p. 494). Fatherhood can extend beyond the definition of a man creating biological offspring through providing sperm (Almeling, 2011), or the belief of a traditional biological father living with his own children, to encompass different contexts (Eggebeen & Knoester, 2001) or a sense of identity. Social scientists define fatherhood as "a set of responsibilities ranging from providing economic support, disciplining children, and serving as a role-model" (Eggebeen & Knoester, 2001, p. 391). Additionally, Pleck (2012) recommends that paternal involvement should include engagement activities, along with social and material indirect care—defined as activities done "for the child but not with the child" (p. 245).

There is scarce research on fathers and their relationships with their adult children. A specific gap in the research involving fathers and their children is what happens when these adult children have a developmental disability. The study thus focuses on exploring the relationships between fathers and their adult children with developmental disabilities according to the fathers themselves. Having a developmental disability can limit self-care, learning, and independent living (Kripke, 2018). Currently, there are estimated to be over seven million people in the US with an Intellectual or Developmental Disability (National Disability Navigator Resource Collaborative, 2020).

Parenthood encompasses roles which are both rewarding and difficult (Senior, 2014). Parents face challenges in raising children and "parenting is more

 | DOI:10.1163/9789004708136_008

stressful today than in prior decades" (Nomaguchi & Milkie, 2020, p. 201). As a child ages into adulthood, the relationship a father has with his child requires adjustments and arrangements (Lye, 1996; Umberson, Pudrovska, & Reczek, 2010). The goals a father may have regarding his child may involve reciprocal communication or a sense of camaraderie through comparable experiences (Roy, 2014a). Although, when a child has an Intellectual and Developmental Disability (IDD), communication may be difficult and establishing camaraderie may not happen as expected. Examples of required adjustments and practices include balancing employment with child-care needs, encouraging participation in opportunities which can promote a child's well-being (e.g., sports or clubs at school), and working out how advanced education or options regarding a child's future can be planned, paid for and successfully executed (Fingerman et al., 2012). Parenting behavior and parent-child relationships can be affected by several contextual factors which can change over the life course. Thus, research on fathering should not be limited to parent-child relationships when children are young (Schoppe-Sullivan & Fagan, 2020). Fatherly love and involvement are not new—but as the Pew Report and other studies have shown—many people in society have changed their definitions and framings of these concepts (Roy, 2014b; Williams, 2008). Fatherhood, once entered, is a lifelong role, and parent-child relationships contain life course expectations, disruptions, adjustments, and varying levels of involvement (Seltzer & Bianchi, 2013; Umberson & Montez, 2010).

This study examined the experiences of mid-life and later-life fathers (age range 46 to 74 years) who have adult children with developmental disabilities, including the challenges they have faced and the resources they have utilized. By interviewing fathers of adult children with developmental disabilities, this study provided insight into the current state of fatherhood in terms of the role of father and father involvement. This study spoke to the two main research questions of: (1) How do fathers understand their involvement in the lives of their adult children with developmental disabilities—to include any changes across the life course? and (2) What supports do fathers utilize and what challenges and constraints do fathers feel they have faced as fathers of adult children with developmental disabilities?

I first review two theoretical perspectives which provided the foundation of this research: life course perspective and disability frameworks, to include relevant empirical research. It is followed by discussing the qualitative methodology used through analyzing fifteen interviews with fathers themselves. Results include finding that some fathers engage in activities with their adult child, whereas other fathers see themselves as having interdependency with their child. The final discussion provides discourse on the major implications of this research as related to sociological theory, and for understanding the resource supports and future directions regarding men who are fathers with adult children with developmental disabilities.

1 Life Course Perspective

A life course framework is built on the premise that people live lives which are socially organized in biological and historical time. The resulting social patterns influence the ways we feel, think, and act (Elder, 1998). Specifically, "life transitions are always part of social trajectories that give them distinctive meaning and form" (Elder, 1998, p. 1). The timing and ordering of transitions come with a constructed meaning. Events can happen out of order, such as returning to school later in life. Events may be considered ill-timed, with war as an example. Lastly, events may be considered as off-timed, such as a change in jobs. When these types of events or transitions happen when not expected or anticipated, adverse effects can occur and can be considered a disruption in a life course. Regardless, various opportunities, constraints, changes and processes, such as parenting and aging, have consequences for individuals (Elder, Johnson, & Crosnoe, 2003).

Individuals do not exist alone in life. One key principle of the life course paradigm is linked lives, which states: "lives are lived interdependently, and social and historical influences are expressed through this network of shared relationships" (Elder, 1998, p. 4). As a result, these social ties become a form of social support, control, and constraint with lives interacting and connecting in influential ways. This life course paradigm can be applied to the meaning of parenthood. For example, a transition in the life of one person can mean a transition in the life of their family member, such as adult children moving back home (Davis, Kim, & Fingerman, 2018). Life course perspective is especially focused on the concept of time, and as life expectancy continues to increase, more parents will potentially require assistance from their children at some point (Fingerman et al., 2010). Fingerman and colleagues (2010) further discuss a life course paradigm in their study of middle-aged adults when they state that parents assist their children until late in life when declines in health may reverse the flow, necessitating parents turning to their children for assistance. This situation of parents continuing to provide assistance to their adult children also remains common (Fingerman, Huo, & Birditt, 2020). Families are likely to share many years in some sort of relationship, more so than in the past, which means fathers and children typically have more opportunities to have relationships across time in their lives (Roy, 2014a).

Living longer means an increase in the possibility of having complex family relationships and with multiple persons. Fatherhood is a role and contains its own dynamics, relationships and characteristics. This role is altered over the life course, and when disruptions occur—such as having an adult child with a disability who does not launch, navigating a return to the original role may be a challenge. Launching refers to the stage of when a child moves out of their parental home (Collischon, Eberl, & Wolbring, 2021). Family Life Cycle Theory suggests that mastery of the skills and milestones in one stage allows an individual to successfully move to the next stage of life (Healthwise Staff, 2020). Coping with a disability can delay these transitions or effect the needed skills for adapting and successfully functioning in another life stage, such as being able to live independently. Additionally, the cultural meanings and structural factors in place influencing the first generation of fathers may not be the same as the factors and constraints which influenced how the son was and is able to father. "Transitions for fathers and children are likely to influence fathers' perceptions of the role" (Stelle & Sheehan, 2011, p. 61). Parenting also involves expectations and predictions and when a child does not meet this expectation, the nature and quality of the relationship is different. This "dis-alignment," or a disruption to the life course, is an area I explored in my research involving fathers and their adult children who have developmental disabilities. The principle of linked lives reminds us that no individual is completely independent (Elder, 1998).

This life course perspective provides added insight into a study of fathers with adult children with developmental disabilities, although few studies have explicitly studied this subject. Marsack and Perry (2018) note how parenting and providing care for a child with a developmental disability (specifically, Autism Spectrum Disorder) means there is not an end to their role as caregiver. People live longer and as a result of the dynamics of linked lives, parents must negotiate a balance of caring for their adult child, maintaining relationships with their other children and family members, and pursuing personal fulfilment for themselves, especially as they enter into old age with their own physical and mental health concerns (Marsack & Perry, 2018).

1.1 *Parenthood and Family Life*

As proposed by a gender as relational approach, studies considering the experiences of fatherhood need to keep in mind social understandings and experiences of motherhood. Schoppe-Sullivan and Fagan (2020) examined literature on fathers over the last twenty years and found one challenge which remains: Research on parenting tends to default to mothers as representative of parenthood within a family. Researchers find mothers spend more time with their children and thus, mark them as the primary caregiver. Even today many people believe mothers are better equipped to care for children than fathers (Parker & Livingston, 2018).

Studies have shown that men being caregivers is overlooked by people in society as it does not always fit with one's traditional perception and understanding of masculinity. As a result, caring masculinity may be disregarded because care and caring are generally associated with women and femininity. However, recasting traditional values into interdependent care-oriented values is a part of caring masculinity. By arguing that traditional roles can be flexible, and by engaging in caregiving or care work, men develop caring forms of masculinities and nurturing identities. It also demonstrates that care values, emotions and masculinities are intertwined (Lee & Lee, 2016).

Studies also show that the care work men provide are important aspects of their role within the family. For fathers, it has been reported that caring for their children helped the fathers become more nurturing and sensitive and that they developed a respect of caregiving (Lee & Lee, 2016). Scholars, such as Aldous, Mulligan and Bjarnason (1998), Fingerman (2001), Eggebeen, Dew, and Knoester (2010), and Roy (2014a), have studied parenthood and found that fathers who provide care for their children reconstruct their concept of fathering through this care. It was also found that their subjective notion of a positive well-being is a beneficial outcome produced through this care. When speaking to parenting children with disabilities, Boström and Broberg (2014) found that fathers had to deal with a disruption in their plans by changing their perspectives and embracing flexibility. These researchers also found that fathers reaped rewards from being involved in the caregiving needs of their child with an IDD, along with feeling that the challenges related to the disability affected their parenthood positively and made them a better parent (Boström & Broberg, 2014).

Caring masculinity can be said to showcase the new and involved father. Hunter, Riggs, and Augoustinos (2017) remind us that fatherly love and involvement is not new, regardless of the packaging or titling. Returning to Schoppe-Sullivan and Fagan (2020), they report an argument that the definition for the role of father is not as clear and understood as what is there for mother. Irrespective of any one explanation of the father role, in today's society-mostly contemporary western society, men are expected to be more involved in caregiving, regardless of the opportunities to explore their nurturing traits (Hunter et al., 2017). Illness, injury, age, a lack of resources, or other events, can be experienced by anyone, thus, increasing their level of dependence (Landes & Settersten, 2019). Furthermore, it is not uncommon for people with a disability to require some type of assistance at some point in time.

In speaking to parenting an adult child with a developmental disability, long-term planning must be considered—for both the parents as they age and for the care of the adult child (Marsack & Perry, 2018).

2 Disability Aspects

This study explored fathers who have an adult child with a developmental disability and therefore, required a grounding in a theoretical and sociological understanding of disability to include the social model of disability and a sociological perspective regarding the body. According to the 106th public law of congress (2000) (Kripke, 2018)—S. 1809/P.L. 106–402 Developmental Disabilities Assistance and Bill of Rights Act of 2000 (US National Archives and Records Administration 2021) a developmental disability is a severe and chronic disability of an individual attributable to a mental and/or physical impairment manifested before an individual reaches the age of 22 years. A developmental disability results in functional limitations in at least three major life activity areas, to include self-care, learning, receptive and expressive language, mobility, the capacity for independent living, and economic self-sufficiency. Lastly, a developmental disability is likely to continue indefinitely and will reflect an individual's need for services, supports and assistance for a lifelong or an extended duration of time (The Association of University Centers on Disabilities, 2000). An Intellectual Disability (ID) replaces the outdated "Mental Retardation" term from the ICD-10 current American medical coding (Tomlinson et al., 2014).

Historically, any perception of someone being not-like-everyone-else, or any perceived type of non-normalness of a body, its parts or functioning process or capacity, to include physical or mental, was considered an illness or a disability (Turner, 2001). This belief transformed into the medical system, with its expanding authority and jurisdiction (Conrad, 2005), emphasizing, or even constructing, a disorder, an illness, sickness, or a lacking, based either on something medical or causing an issue related to the medical. The medical was synonymous with biological, which then gave rise to medicalization—"the creation of new medical categories" (Conrad, 2005, p. 3). If the disease or disorder was placed into a medical context, then it could be fixed, but also implied it needed fixed, making medical intervention imperative for proper functioning (Turner, 2001).

People with disabilities have bodies which need medical care, just as all bodies should utilize a combination of care factors. Utilizing a medical model does not imply sickness is a requirement, however, though bodies are evolutionary and biological (Turner, 1991). Additionally, mental and developmental are a part of embodiment, also requiring a medical continuum of care (Verbrugge & Jette, 1994). Defining disability as illness makes for a vague explanation. Are physical disabilities the same as mental disabilities because they fall under the umbrella term of "disabilities" or should we even put mental in the same medical model where physical may fall (Chang & Leung, 2020; Oliver, 1996)? "Developmental disabilities" has its own distinct and separate definition and criteria, to include aetiologies which can affect and lead to differences in behaviors and personalities of individuals (Ricci & Hodapp, 2003).

The medical can provide the causal explanation—the "why," which can then help with understanding the processes or potential manifestations and outcomes of genetic or environmental aetiologies—the "in what ways." However, the resulting understandings, adaptations and modifications are social (Zola, 1972). There are physiological differences in the brain for someone with a developmental disability. Additionally, as stated above, mental processing, behavioral manifestations and aging, along with personality nuances, are directly linked to brain physiology and genetic aetioloies (Ricci & Hodapp, 2003) and are beyond resulting from solely psychological or social factors. Abilities and strengths in one area may also mask challenges in another area. For example, deficits in hearing does not mean cognitive disjunction, or vice-versa. The goal of health care for a patient with a developmental disability is to improve their well-being and function and, therefore, it may not be necessary to change any specific characteristic of the patient (Kripke, 2018). Even though a disability may likely be attributed to a medical reasoning or genetic aetiology, participating in a community setting may contain unrelated challenges, which are social reasonings, such as others not being welcoming toward an individual with a disability. Socially, which is separate from the medical or a physical equipment need, a community site can be modified or adjusted so a disabled person can participate and contribute in a welcoming and accommodating manner.

Writings by sociologists have discussed the body and in a myriad of ways. Charmaz (1995) writes about "experiencing an altered body" (p. 659). Turner (2001) provides, "Who I am cannot be separated from how I am embodied" (p. 254). Zola (1991) writes about his own body's experiences, as well as how his perceptions changed in regard to societal viewpoints over time. Nowakowski (2016), to name another example, discusses how a chronic illness can lead one to be labeled, with assumptions made about behavior and beauty. Keeping the body in the disability definition means that any processes involving the body are subject to illness and must be treated (Kripe, 2018). Molton and Yorkston (2017) discuss aging with a disability, naming resilience, flexibility and appropriate medical care, as indicators of success. Verbrugge and Yang (2002) remind their readers that "disability and aging interweave over the life course" (p. 266). Additionally, the life expectancy of people with developmental disabilities is starting to reach that of the general population, having increased from living an average age of only nineteen years in the 1930s (Kripke, 2018).

Disability is a limitation, restriction or lack of ability to perform the activities considered normal for one's role in society (Oliver, 1996; Verbrugge & Jette, 1994). However, disability can be contested in its significance, origins, production and boundaries (Coleman-Fountain and McLaughlin, 2013). A sociomedical model leans toward the meshing of two parts: one, how a condition affects the body (or part of the body) and its functioning, and two, the related and effecting personal or environmental factors involved (Verbrugge & Jette, 1994). Twenty-five years later, research continues to remind us that persons with disabilities can be healthy because, again, a disability is not an illness. Plus, the neurodiversity and social models view disability as a natural part of life (Kripke, 2018).

The label itself of the sociomedical path keeps the body involved, thus maintaining the medical as the dominant half. The definition of disability above implies the body is minimally involved. Truth be told, the body must remain involved because with the body and through the body is how one interacts with the environment. Regardless of how society tries to remove barriers, the fact remains that it is sometimes the individual body itself which is the barrier. Society looks at what a body does and can do. In other words, individuals seek a body which interacts in expected ways. Reaching a goal of success and of being valued (McLaughlin, 2017) comes with care and attitude, whether self-care and self-sufficiency, or care from others.

Disability is not the same as illness and Parsons (1975) questioned if illness could mean the same as disabled. Albrecht (2010) writes about trying to separate sick from disabled, implying that the disabled do not get sick, though "most disabled individuals are dealing with multiple disabilities and comorbidities at the same time" (p. 204). In this case, the medical model needs to be kept in the forefront of research and discussion. However, one cannot focus on one area of a person with complete disregard for another characteristic or encompassed role. People with developmental disabilities also get sick and require medical care (Videlefsky et al., 2019; Kripe, 2018).

By removing social problems away from the religious and moral scrutiny into a medical arena judgments continue to be made, but instead, in the name of health (Zola, 1972). The medical world influences people to adopt a goal of doing all you can to feel better, look better and function better. Some could argue that labeling is just a medical processing (Coleman-Fountain et al., 2013) but Goffman connected labeling to stigma of persons with disabilities because it was used as a judgment about value and worth. This stigmatizing became a way to normalize institutional discrimination in ways to access resources and opportunities (Lucas, Greenberg, & Beavan, 2017). Stigma and judgments involve attitudes which can translate into low expectations for parents to "successfully" raise their children with disabilities or that parents are to feel emotionally encumbered raising them. Challenges and burdens are to be faced solely by the parents and family, making support and appreciation for time, expenses and tasks inadequate and misunderstood (Green, 2007).

One highlight in combining the theories of life course perspective and disability frameworks, is that the presence of disability has profound effects on individuals, as well as those close to these individuals. As a result, disability "play[s] an important role in the lives of most Americans" (Lucas, Greenberg, & Beavan, 2017, p. 1). Disability also shapes social interactions. For parents, parenting behavior and relationships with their children are affected by numerous contextual factors, including social (Schoppe-Sullivan & Fagan, 2020). Parenting challenges, stressors and rewards take different forms across their life course (Nomaguchi & Milkie, 2020), with family member roles and meanings in later life being different than from earlier in life. How men construct paternal identity is the basis for their self-conception as a father and for fathering, and thus, creates motivation for their fathering behavior (Pleck, 2012). Rarely is a life course framework linked to disabilities, especially regarding linked lives or disrupted life course. One strength of this project is that combination.

3 Methodology

3.1 *Research Design and Data Procedures*

This study involved fatherhood and its effects surrounding parenting their adult children who have a developmental disability. A qualitative approach was employed using in-depth interviews. My main research inquiries addressed: (1) How do fathers understand their involvement in the lives of their adult children with developmental disabilities—to include any changes across the life course? and (2) What supports do fathers utilize and what challenges and constraints do fathers feel they have faced as fathers of adult children with disabilities? Approval for recruiting, conducting interviews, and the data collection and analysis was granted by the Institutional Review Board (IRB) through The University of Alabama at Birmingham.

I argue that my research questions related to how fathers envision their involvement level with the adult children with an IDD is best viewed through a qualitative lens, specifically through in-depth interviews with fathers themselves. Researchers explore the perspective, thoughts, and feelings the research subjects or participants themselves hold (Charmaz, 2006; Babbie, 1995). Qualitative methodology is a way to explore social properties that result from interactions between individuals (Bryman, 2016), along with how cultural contexts and social conditions influence meanings and experiences (Braun & Clark, 2006). For this reason, I used the qualitative method of in-depth interviews to collect and analyze fathers' own narratives and perspectives, having conducted face-to-face interviews using a semi-structured questionnaire. As every father has their own story to tell, conducting real-time interviews allowed for an elaboration of the stories told and an encouragement to share pertinent details.

The selection criteria for a father to be able to participate in this study included if a man considered himself to be a father of an adult child with a developmental disability and co-resided with that child at the time of the interview. The goal was to interview fathers of adult children who were diagnosed with a type of developmental disability. While an IQ test score is no longer used as the sole criteria for a diagnosis, it may be part of a series of standardized tests and mental abilities for adaptive functioning (APA, 2021). However, as children who tested on the autism spectrum usually have a form of IDD, if they were of the appropriate age, their fathers qualified as participants in the study.

Recruitment was conducted via areas in three states: East Coast, Midwest and Deep South. I recruited most heavily in a Deep South region. In recruiting, I visited community agencies in-person where services were provided for persons with an IDD, along with sending emails to contact persons recommended to me. Additionally, I sent the recruitment fliers for them to be able to distribute to their individuals and post on their social media sites and other places they deemed appropriate. I received referrals through Special Olympics—an organization which provides sports training and athletic competition to individuals with intellectual disabilities (Special Olympics, 2021). Other fathers who participated in this project were referrals through other local support resources and settings, and from mutual acquaintances.

Fifteen fathers participated in interviews. All names are changed to preserve confidentiality. Fathers ranged in age from 46 years to 74 years. Twelve fathers had sons and three had daughters. The age range of the adult children was 18 to 40 years. All adult children had always resided in the home with the parents. Two fathers were stepfathers and all fathers were married to the mother of the adult child with an IDD. Of the diagnoses identified, nine had a diagnosis of Down Syndrome and/or Autism. Down Syndrome is a condition in which a person is has an extra chromosome. This additional genetic material changes how a baby's brain and body develops, causing both mental and physical challenges for the baby (Centers for Disease Control and Prevention, 2021; National Down Syndrome Society, 2021). Autism is a lifelong developmental disability, typically starting in childhood, affecting a person's social skills and self-regulation (Autism Society, 2024).

Interviews averaged about an hour and were conducted in a variety of places with most having taken place in the father's home. Interviews were conducted using a semi-structured guide which allowed for flexibility, expansion, and probing in specific areas appropriate to the topic and specific research participant. The basics of the formal interview covered functionality and abilities of the adult child, a brief account about how a diagnosis and services were acquired and which ones were needed, along with daily activities ("Tell me about a typical day regarding you and your child"). Conversation turned toward day programming and employment, or other events or activities in which the adult child might occupy his or her time. The section to address relationship involved questions directly asking for a descriptor, parenting style, or the relationship dad had with his own father. Asking about what supports were utilized frequently led into comments about what supports exist in the area in which they live or have lived, along with what is needed or recommended.

Analysis of the data was done using an abductive research strategy (Timmermans and Tavory, 2012). Abduction is explanatory hunches based on clues. It "explores the most plausible explanation from an array of possibilities" (Saldaña, 2011, p. 94). Abduction blends inductive and deductive reasoning. It refers to the "process of generating social scientific accounts from social actors' accounts" (Ong, 2012, p. 7) and the participants' perspectives (Bryman, 2016). It gives attention to the meanings, motives and interpretations actors use in their lives. Coding is the link between data collection and developing theory to explain it (Charmaz, 2014), along with serving to note what is happening in the data, remaining open to interpretation. Focused coding follows and entails identifying the most common themes and which ones make the most sense for categorizing the data; thus, what can be considered as representing the real-world phenomena (Bryman, 2016). The final stage of analysis was reached when it was found that no new themes were emerging from the data, with this determination being the definition for theoretical saturation (Charmaz, 2014; Bryman, 2016).

4 Results

Using Life Course and Disability as the main theoretical frameworks guiding this research, the following section will provide a discourse from the analysis about two of the themes—"An Inextricable Link" and "Supports"—which emerged from the data. First, using the theory of Life Course, particularly the concepts of Disrupted Lives and Linked Lives as a foundation, this study observed fathers incorporating their family life and children into their life course. Though the initial knowledge regarding an atypical and unexpected diagnosis and prognosis may have spoken to a disruption in the life course, these fathers did not interpret their lives as being disrupted by a diagnosis made to their child. Rather, these respondents stayed their intended course and, to do so, linked their child's life into their own, with some fathers continuing this linkage into their future through an interdependency. Thus, "an inextricable link." The theme of "supports" produced three subthemes—wife, job, and religious faith. A few husbands provided examples of when and how their wives were a source of support. A few men specifically stated their job or working was a source of support for them, with some fathers having already retired. Lastly, several men pointedly identified that their religious faith or their church was a source of support for them.

All of the fathers interviewed could have been placed in almost any one subtheme or in multiple subthemes simultaneously. Additionally, the subthemes discussed below are not distinct nor mutually exclusive labels for characterizing fatherhood, nor for fathers who have adult children with a developmental disability. In Section 5, how fathers fit across and between subthemes will be described.

4.1 *An Inextricable Link*

Under the main theoretical frameworks of Life Course and Disability, I found that men in this study perceived their lives as not disrupted by the presence of their adult child who had a developmental disability. Instead, they still saw their lives as closely and indistinguishably linked to their adult child. This linking was seen primarily through daily activities. Fathers' support of participation in activities was demonstrated by providing transportation to and from their adult child's job site, assisting the adult child with learning skills toward independence, such as with tasks related to laundry, or accompanying the adult child to sports events in which the adult child was involved. Fathers who themselves do paid work outside the home trust their adult child is safe and gaining or practicing skills in independence through the child's own day programming, whether community employment, a structured day programming environment or even being at home. Fathers who are retired did not readily express their preferred activities, instead indicated finding satisfaction through engaging in activities with their child, with examples of combined activities being civic organizations and sports-related events.

One example of a father and son living linked lives is Gerald and his son Sam. Gerald is 74 and retired. His son, Sam, is 38, and he reports he was diagnosed around the age of five as "Educatably Mentally Retarded"—Mentally Retarded but able to learn skills related to school and daily living. During son Sam's childhood, Gerald talked about his involvement in his son's education and childhood activities, which also included sports and Boy Scouts.

Gerald provided an unanticipated example of how his life is inextricable linked to Sam's when he started talking about his son's health. He shared, "Well, he's picking up adult diseases now. He's diabetic. But no, I didn't anticipate any of that because mentally he's about eight or nine or ten years old. So only physically has he aged, not mentally." When Gerald was asked about retirement, he said, 'I'm going to hang around with Sam.' And that's about what we do. He goes everywhere with me."

When Gerald went to military-related organizations and places, he would take Sam and they welcomed him. "They just loved him. He's got quite a fan club. Everybody knows him. They don't know me from Adam but they know him. 'He's not your son, you're his dad. I'm his dad.' That's what I tell people." He further shared, "I've learned more from him than I've ever been able to teach him…My whole attitude towards people changed watching him interact with people. And I am more willing to go up to strangers now and just introduce myself and carry-on conversations. And it's fun. And I learned that from him… And because of him, I have gotten involved in a lot of activities."

Another example of father and adult child sharing "an inextricable link" in their linked lives is Keith, aged 64 and medically retired, and his son Scott, age 25, who was diagnosed with Autism when he was a toddler. Keith expressed joy in his son. Specifically, "When Scott came, I realized it's time to forget about me completely…I've enjoyed being Scott's dad most days…It's the biggest thrill I have ever had." These sentiments of Keith regarding Scott indicate that Keith does not feel Scott is a disruption to his life course.

In describing events and activities, Keith named "the big four" activities: church, Civil War re-enacting, NASCAR, and trains. These activities were stated for both of them, not just listed as what Scott liked to do. Thus, combined interests and activities proving that Keith's life is linked to Scott's. Keith expressed the socialness of Scott and that he enjoys watching Scott's interactions. "We go to an event. And when he gets to the event, he disappears for the first 45 minutes. He's off somewhere…talking to some of his buds that he knows…And I get more questions when he's not there than when he is there."

Keith made additional comments regarding fathering Scott, and these comments provide the story of their lives being linked. As Scott came to be accepted and then even became an individual member of his own standing, Keith was still considered a member. However, the role of father-with-son turned into two friends or even son-with-father. Consequently, the pride Keith has for his son is heard in the sharing he did, along with the how lives were not only not disrupted but linked. There is also a goal that they and their lives will remain linked, using their shared enjoyment of NASCAR and Civil War re-enactment, among other activities, as their common bonds.

Other fathers interviewed shared the activities in which they engaged with their child, but these two above discussed multiple activities across multiple realms, to include civic, church-related, sports-related, social, and child's employment. The fathers in this subtheme were also supportive of the programming in which their child was engaged and assisted their child with learning skills toward independence. Again, fathers did not express that their child was a disruption to their living with having their adult child with them. Instead, they enjoyed a closeness with their adult child through participating together in activities, whether more major activities, such as a community event, or through daily living tasks, such as driving to work.

4.2 *Supports*

Another major theme which emerged in my research under the main theoretical frameworks of Life Course and Disability involves support. Support was further divided into three subthemes—wife, job, and religious faith. One aspect of Life Course Theory is that it entails interactions among individuals. These social ties and connections are a form of social support (Elder, 1998). Additionally, within a family, its members may be a primary resource for other family members. Thomas, Liu and Umberson (2017) write from their research how parenthood can "increase social integration leading to greater emotional support and a sense of belonging" (p. 4), along with finding that parents tend to provide instrumental and financial support to their adult children. Additionally, social ties, such as those which can promote emotional well-being and physical health, are also protective against stress effects (Thoits, 2011). Results from these ties include a sense of mastery, a feeling of belonging, and a greater level of self-esteem.

Related to having a child with a developmental disability, Davys and colleagues (2016), in their study of existing research, found that fathers who seek out information regarding their child's situation may be done both as a need and as a coping strategy, with knowledge leading to a sense of empowerment. Because fathers "are less likely than mothers to seek social or emotional support" (Boström & Broberg, 2014, p. 811), other sources of support may be found through employment which can provide "material, social and psychological resources" (Nomaguchi & Milkie, 2020, p. 204).

A final point regarding supports father may utilize, involve religion. One's religion may involve their religious faith, their attendance at religious-based places of worship, or a combination of both. Koenig (2008) lays out discourse that religious people need and use fewer health care services because they are heathier and are more likely to have family members to care for them, along with having greater social support. Other resources available to members of religious communities may involve instrumental aid (goods and services), information regarding agencies or support groups, and formal programs related to providing assistance to those in need (Ellison & George, 1994).

4.2.1 Wives

Husbands identifying wives as their source of support included three fathers. One father, Nick, when directly asked about his coping skills, simply stated, "Probably just mostly talking to [wife]. "Another father, Oliver, when asked, shared, "I don't feel like I've had to have a lot of coping skills really, because my wife has dealt with a lot of the sort of day-to-day stuff." Isaac also identified his wife as a source of support with, "I was relying on my wife because she's a great mother. And I knew she would be. So I'm really riding her coat tails."

4.2.2 Job

Switching to work and employment as a source of support for fathers, Benjamin stated, "The kids, the kids keeps me going." Benjamin is a coach for junior high school aged children and what he said emphasizes how important coaching is to him. Eli, a stepfather who said he loves his job, commented about using it as a way to role model for his stepson. He emphasized working when he told him, "Dude, you don't have a better role model than a guy like me. I go to work every day. Every day where's this guy go? Who's not sitting around the house playing video games every day? This guy. Where am I? I'm at work." Another father, Albert, shared about his line of work, "I took, chose a profession that I chose so that I'd never have to quit working. I love to hunt and fish. I love to write and I love to shoot photography."

4.2.3 Religious Faith

Nine fathers shared in some way how their religious faith or church provided a source of support for them, including a few who had also identified another area of support they utilize. One father, Michael, shared, "we've had a lot of ups and downs in our family over the years. I guess, of course, my faith in Christ has, has been a big, big part of that. Just seeing that God's in control and realizing that every situation that you know, you can learn more about yourself, and through the various things that happen."

In naming specific ways in which a religious-based place of worship—church—has provided a tangible service, Albert, mentioned above, reported, "One thing that's really helped us a lot is here at this church…They have a class for kids with special needs…and we're able to go to church together, which before we weren't able to do…We feel like they take care of him just like family does." Faith is a part of Carl's belief system saying his family goes to church together as a family. He also offered, when asked about his mental health, "My wife and I are pretty heavily involved in her church, in small groups, and we found that that's the best way to keep us sort of grounded spiritually and from a mental health standpoint."

Isaac discussed faith as part of what influences his fathering skills when he shared, "I think a lot of it has to do with our Christian faith, to be honestly with you. I find that people of Christian faith, especially if they're serious practitioners, if you will, probably tend to be more like the way I'm doing it. More traditional, more engaged, a little more structured, a little more teaching, you know, that sort of thing. That's what I've observed."

Jim, when asked about his coping resources, talked about his faith and his wife. First, "I have the spiritual gift of faith, by the way, which I know He's [God] going to see it through. I just have to. I just know that." Then, regarding his wife, when talking about his daughter with IDD, "Whatever Mama says, she's like this. Ain't that a blessing. Thank God she's got a good mama."

Keith also discussed his faith when he revealed, "My wife brought me to Christ. My wife made a Christian of me back when we first got married. And I rebelled against all of it. When [Scott] got here, all of a sudden I realized God was toughening that faith to where it would work for me…And He [God] put him here to show me that there is something more than fat old me in the equation."

While several fathers talked about their religious beliefs and in having faith, few stated they had ever participated in a men's groups, father's group, or in any type of support group. Some named their wives as to whom they would talk as a source of support, though revealed no details. Some made comments about an aspect of their job which offered benefit, such as social interactions. And some fathers either overtly stated they did not feel they had used, nor needed, a source of support or a coping resource.

5 Discussion

The emphasis of this study was to explore the relationships between fathers and their adult children who have been diagnosed with a developmental disability, advancing our understanding of this understudied topic within medical and family sociology. This study focused on two theoretical frameworks—Life Course and Disability—and focused on two research aims. These aims were to address the ways fathers understand their involvement with their adult children, and what supports fathers state they have utilized and recommend, along with what challenges and constraints fathers felt they have faced as fathers of adult children with developmental disabilities.

Through qualitative interviewing with fathers with adult children with a developmental disability, results included fathers who engage in activities with their adult child, along with fathers who have an interdependency with their child. Results also found fathers taking on a protector and provider role by wanting to keep their child safe and at home. The end but basic outcome was that fathers frequently use multiple ways to show care and involvement in the lives of their family and with their adult child, identifying their wives or their religious faith as their coping mechanism, or saying none was needed.

Based on these results, I identified implications for our sociological understandings of fathers with adult children with developmental disabilities. These implications were developed through recognizing how my results intersected with previous research and existing theoretical frameworks and provide important insight into future research needed in these areas.

5.1 *Community Involvement: Life Course and Activities*

The first implication is regarding life course with linked lives and disrupted lives. People have connections with others, which become their social ties and the influences for how people feel supported, controlled and constrained. As a result, these interactions, opportunities, and changes have consequences for individuals (Elder, 1998; Elder, Johnson, & Crosnoe, 2003). A life course framework, as explained by Elder (1998), is built on the premise that people live lives interdependently with others. Their connections to others are influential sources of both strain and support. Throughout one's life, events and transitions may or may not happen. Some are expected, but when they are not or do not happen, a disruption to the life course occurs.

People being connected to others, and thus having linked lives, was illustrated through the activities fathers did with their adult child and other family members. Some of the fathers were excited to share about the activities they did with their child, along with some talking more about activities they have engaged in together more recently. These activities included driving their child to and from an event or employment, sporting events, either watching them on television or with the child participating in a team, civic activities, church-related endeavors, social pursuits, and even national events, examples being marathons and National Down Syndrome conferences.

Besides activities outside of the home, many fathers in telling their stories talked about what the adult child does at home, even to include watching television and video gaming. The most common example identified was helping out with household responsibilities, as having a developmental disability can be a challenge for self-care and independent living (Kripke, 2018). Some fathers, more so the younger ones, want their child to gain life skills so launching can potentially occur, even if reached later than expected or desired. On the other hand, older fathers talked about having their adult child help with chores and household activities but with more of the implication that it was good to have an additional helping hand in the house. And therefore, any work on living skills was not for the purpose of moving out.

No father stated that there had been disruptions in their lives with regard to their child. However, needing to make adjustments of any sort, including an initial diagnosing of a child, is a type of disruption. None of the fathers interviewed reported that their adult child had significant behavioral issues. Additionally, fathers did not dwell or focus on their child's health or physical needs as being problematic. Adjustments had been made, and fathers, when discussing future plans, had provisions in place to cover these needs as the adult child aged.

In summary, "involvement" meant "including" the child who had an IDD in activities in the home and/or out of the home. All the fathers I interviewed were married to the child's mother resulting in mom being a source of assistance and schedule-arranging. Serving as a reminder, Marsack and Perry (2018) reported that parenting and providing care for a child with a developmental disability means the caregiving role does not end and must be balanced in with other relationships and responsibilities.

5.2 *Faith and Religion as Supports*

Another implication encompasses faith and religion. Putnam (2000) reports that religion has "traditionally been a central fount of American community life and health" (p. 79). Wilcox (2004) writes that in a general sense, religion has a "pro-social effect on family behavior" (p. 104), including on fathers being associated with higher levels of affection and involvement. Even though some recruiting was through churches which housed programs for families who had a family member with an IDD, only three fathers specifically came from this recruitment. However, when asking about coping skills and resources, most of these fathers shared aspects of their faith, even if "faith" was not a direct response to the question about coping.

One article reported that research done over the last twenty years has found that fathers who rated religion as important in their lives had a positive relationship with their children, also putting forth effort into the relationship (Kim

& Swan, 2019). The point made by these authors speaks to the fathers in my study because in backing up twenty years, the adult children of these fathers were between infancy and emerging adulthood ages, and thus, in their formative years. Additionally, religion and church may have been a resource utilized by fathers directly or indirectly (Wilcox, 2004).

Nine of the fathers I interviewed readily stated church or faith was a source of support for them. Four others mentioned religion or church in some way by either stating they sometimes attend services, sharing knowledge about a respite program through a local church, or being referred to this study through a church-related environment. This project was not about religiosity but a future direction could inquire about how faith has correlated with a father's sense of resilience or in what ways religion or church has been a resource over his life course. Putnam (2000) reports that "churches have been and continue to be important institutional providers of social services" (p. 67).

5.3 *Structural Constraints*

A third implication regarding fatherhood involves the role of structural constraints. While the fathers I interviewed did not speak directly to these constraints, instead providing more of a positive narrative, constraints were implicit in the analysis and are highlighted below. These constraints involve age, de-institutionalization, and supports.

5.3.1 Age

Looking at the age range of fathers in this study, which spanned from 46 to 74 years, no clear distinctions could be made based on older versus younger. Two of the oldest fathers still worked in a job setting. Three of the youngest six fathers wanted their adult child to launch, talking that it was almost expected or that they will push the child toward it. However, the other three in this grouping had children who were lower functioning and needed assistance with their daily living skills. Because of this lower functioning level, it cannot be assumed that these fathers were the model for the new and involved father, or even intensive fathering. Their children simply needed more intensive care. Subsequently, "today's fathers" may really mean fathers younger in age or fathers of young children, whether or not they have a child with a developmental disability. As this study was about fathers with adult children, projections about fathers who are young in age or who have young children are beyond the scope of this study.

5.3.2 De-institutionalization and Public Health

Seltzer and colleagues (2011) state parents have only recently been living in a time of de-institutionalization. Thus, they are the first cohort of parents to be negotiating caregiving and be provided with resources and supports to help with their child's needs. Also to be navigating having an individual with an IDD become a productive and involved member of society. However, these parents may also be experiencing health issues due to those pressures, especially as they themselves age and struggle with making sure their child's future is secured along with securing care for their own potential care needs. "The fact that more than one-third of adults with IDD continue to live with their parents through the time when the parents are in their mid-sixties underscores the high probability of continued co-residence" (Seltzer et al., 2011, p. 13). Therefore, these researchers advocate for more public health services to include in-home family supports and respite opportunities. A decade later, Nomaguchi and Milkie (2020) remind readers that policy making needs to reflect the financial and emotional needs parents face while raising children across life stages. While it has been shown that two factors which attribute to adults with developmental disabilities living healthier and longer lives are fewer people living in an institution and improved access to medical care (Videlefsky et al., 2019), the mortality rates for this population could further improve if "public health policies were more focused on interventions" (Gilbert, 2019, p. 2).

5.3.3 Supports and Resources

This study did not request fathers discuss all the potential supports, both private and government-related, which they explored or to which they might have access. Individuals with developmental disabilities are subject to the local and state qualification requirements for services and resources which they may or may not be able to access due to location and other factors, such as transportation, skills and ability levels, and waiting lists. In terms of support groups in which fathers could participate, many did not know of any or made comments related to not believing a support group would be beneficial. No one commented about having had individual counseling, nor even marriage counseling, even as a form of assistance to navigating their situation of having a child with an IDD. However, some fathers did say they would tell other fathers to explore and seek out potential resources. Depending on a researcher's area of focus, a future direction could involve a more pointed exploration regarding supports and resources. For example, what options exist in what geographical area or in what ways a men's support group provides emotional support.

In summation, de-institutionalization and access to services for individuals with a developmental disability, in general, have improved over the decades, but policies need to continue to change and evolve to reflect current times and the needs of families. Additionally, supports and resources need to, first, exist in areas where they are lacking, and second, adjust and progress in areas where they do exist so families can access what they need. Community education and public health communication are avenues which can lead families to be made aware of resources from which they could benefit.

6 Limitations

Despite the strengths of this study, the findings should also be interpreted with an awareness of limitations. Trying to fit fathers into mutually exclusive categories or groupings is difficult for the simple reason that fatherhood is not just made up of one definition or one point in time. These fathers were a rather homogeneous group. Specifically, they were all married to the mother of the adult child with an IDD, and all the adult children resided in their family home and always had. This homogeneity is a potential limit to this study but also enforces the point that the traits and beliefs of fathers are interwoven and can be messy to untangle.

None of the adult children had reported, nor diagnosed, behavioral issues. Additionally, hardly any adult child had detrimental medical concerns. Separately, as this study contained only a few female adult children, future studies should remedy this deficit. Including more female adult children could show if fathers treated their female children differently than their male children. For example, it is difficult to discern if fathers of daughters—in general—do not believe daughters should participate in sports-related activities or if fathers tend to leave it up to the mother to decide in which activities a daughter should participate. All of the fathers in this study were involved in their child's life. Fathers who are not involved, regardless of reason, may be more difficult to find. Not to mention if they are willing to participate and be interviewed for a study about this topic. The reasons a father may have for lack of involvement can range from relationship factors with the mother of the child to policy and service parameters at a time and place surrounding the child and his or her circumstances. Recruiting in institutional settings involves other requirements which time and future studies can follow. Summarizing, who is interviewed and what responses are received will change the nature of the analysis and thus, the outcome and results. What follows is a discussion of potential outcomes.

This project offered a glimpse into the lives of fathers who have an adult child with a developmental disability. A study of a larger magnitude may reach fathers who have adult children in residential settings, or who have a range of physical or mental health concerns, to include behavioral challenges. Additionally, expanding this study to find more adult children who require assistance with their activities of daily living, along with a wider range of functioning and ability levels, will yield other coping skills and possibly a wider array of answers about how to facilitate involvement. Also to services utilized and needed.

This research project in medical sociology was a cross-sectional study meant to capture information through one-time interviews. Of course, a longitudinal study would answer some questions that these fathers did not provide. A snapshot in time a cross-sectional study captures relies on memory. Individuals "include the most meaningful and important aspects of shared experiences into their life stories" (de Vries et al., 2017, p. 58). Memories can lose details over time and along with the factors and influences on how a situation was created, may become less impactful in the retelling and with time. Additionally, "human memory is not objective or always reliable" (Smith & Sparkes, 2016, p. 118). Fathers may have wanted to showcase involvement and therefore, putting their best foot forward in talking to me may have meant a deliberate attempt to *not* reveal certain feelings or situations. In many cases I was younger than my interview subject. I am also not a father. These factors may have led some fathers to not discuss personal stressors or to not reveal certain thoughts or actions.

Individuals with a developmental disability are living longer. Consequently, research regarding mortality factors, quality of life, and end of life will need a continued evaluation for best practices in navigating the changing characteristics of this population. Having worked in the field of developmental disabilities, and more specifically as a supervisor for group homes, there remains a need for community integration, resources for positive supports, and policy adjustment pertaining to services for individuals with an IDD and their families.

7 Conclusion

The definition and framings society dictates for how a father should be involved with his child have not remained permanent through time. Fatherly love and involvement seem to change in its definitions and framings. Father-child relationships require adjustments and arrangements which are influenced by several factors and change over the life course. Having a child with a developmental disability is one such factor. Although parenting remains a challenging role with family ties affecting physical and psychological well-being, these ties also provide a source of positive support. Fathers may find that embracing traits related to caring masculinity (e.g., valuing emotions, increasing interdependency) benefit their health and well-being.

Based on this study, fathers derive health benefits from being involved in the lives of their adult children and utilizing supports and resources. This involvement and which supports can be used will change over the life course. For example, retirement may allow for exploring other pursuits and new friendships for both father and adult child. Both fathers and their adult children with developmental disabilities are living longer. Thus, these relationships will consist of more opportunities for teaching and learning from each other. Other opportunities include engaging in mutually enjoyable activities and encouraging each other to take care of themselves and each other for maximizing health and health behaviors.

References

Albrecht, G. L. (2010). The sociology of disability: Historical foundations and future directions. In C. E. Bird, P. Conrad, & S. Timmermans (Eds.), *Handbook of medical sociology* (pp. 192–209). Vanderbilt University Press.

Aldous, J., Mulligan, G. M., & Bjarnason, T. (1998). Fathering over time: What makes the difference? *Journal of Marriage and the Family* 60(4), 809–820. https://doi.org/10.2307/353626

Almeling, R. (2011). *Sex cells: The medical market for eggs and sperm.* University of California Press.

American Psychiatric Association. (2021). *What is intellectual disability?* Retrieved June 19, 2021, from https://www.psychiatry.org/patients-families/intellectual-disability/what-is-intellectual-disability

The Association of University Centers on Disabilities. (2000). *106th public law of Congress.* Retrieved November 28, 2020, from https://www.aucd.org/docs/urc/dd_act_011907.pdf

Autism Society. (2024). *Autism spectrum disorder.* Retrieved August 16, 2024, from https://autismsociety.org/the-autism-experience/

Babbie, E. (1995). *The practice of social research* (7th ed.). Wadsworth Publishing Company.

Boström, P. K., & Broberg, M. (2014). Openness and avoidance—A longitudinal study of fathers of children with intellectual disability. *Journal of Intellectual Disability Research, 58*(9), 810–821. https://doi.org/10.1111/jir.12093

Braun, V., & Clarke, V. (2006). Using thematic analysis in psychology. *Qualitative Research in Psychology, 3*(2), 77–101. https://doi.org/10.1191/1478088706qp063oa

Bryman, A. (2016). *Social research methods* (5th ed.). Oxford University Press.

Centers for Disease Control and Prevention. (2021). *Facts about Down Syndrome.* Retrieved June 29, 2021, from https://www.cdc.gov/ncbddd/birthdefects/downsyndrome.html

Chan, K. K. S., & Leung, D. C. K. (2020). Linking child autism to parental depression and anxiety: Mediating the roles of enacted and felt stigma. *Journal of Autism and Developmental Disorders, 2020*, 1–11. https://doi.org/10.1007/s10803-020-04557-6

Charmaz, K. (1995). The body, identity, and self: Adapting to impairment. *The Sociological Quarterly, 36*(4), 657–680. https://doi.org/10.1111/j.1533-8525.1995.tb00459.x

Charmaz, K. (2006). *Constructing grounded theory: A practical guide through qualitative analysis*. Sage.

Charmaz, K. (2014). *Constructing grounded theory* (2nd ed.). Sage.

Coleman-Fountain, E., & McLaughlin, J. (2013). The interactions of disability and impairment. *Social Theory & Health, 11*(2), 133–150. https://doi.org/10.1057/sth.2012.21

Conrad, P. (2005). The shifting engines of medicalization. *Journal of Health and Social Behavior, 46*(1), 3–14.

Davis, E. M., Kim, K., & Fingerman, K. L. (2018). Is an empty nest best? Coresidence with adult children and parental marital quality before and after the Great Recession. *The Journals of Gerontology: Series B, 73*(3), 372–381. https://doi.org/10.1093/geronb/gbw022

Davys, D., Mitchell, D., & Martin, R. (2017). Fathers of people with intellectual disability: A review of the literature. *Journal of Intellectual Disabilities, 21*(2), 175–196. https://doi.org/10.1177/1744629516650129

de Vries, B., LeBlanc, A. J., Frost, D. M., Alston-Stepnitz, E., Stephenson, R., & Woodyatt, C. R. (2017). The relationship timeline: A method for the study of shared lived experiences in relational contexts. *Advances in Life Course Research, 32*, 55–64. https://doi.org/10.1016/j.alcr.2016.07.002

Eggebeen, D. J., Dew, J., & Knoester, C. (2010). Fatherhood and men's lives at middle age. *Journal of Family Issues, 31*(1), 113–130. https://doi.org/10.1177/0192513X09341446

Eggebeen, D. J., & Knoester, C. (2001). Does fatherhood matter for men? *Journal of Marriage and Family, 63*(2), 381–393. https://doi.org/10.1111/j.1741-3737.2001.00381.x

Elder Jr., G. H. (1998). The life course as developmental theory. *Child Development, 69*(1), 1–12.

Elder, G. H., Kirkpatrick Johnson, M., & Crosnoe, R. (2003). The emergence and development of life course theory. In J. T. Mortimer & M. J. Shanahan (Eds.), *Handbook of the life course* (pp. 3–19). Springer. https://doi.org/10.1007/978-0-306-48247-2_1

Ellison, C. G., & George, L. K. (1994). Religious involvement, social ties, and social support in a Southeastern community. *Journal for the Scientific Study of Religion*, 33(1), 46–61. https://doi.org/10.2307/1386636

Fingerman, K. (2001). A distant closeness: Intimacy between parents and their children in later life. *Generations, 25*(2), 26–33.

Fingerman, K. L., Cheng, Y.-P., Wesselmann, E. D., Zarit, S., Furstenberg, F., & Birditt, K. S. (2012). Helicopter parents and landing pad kids: Intense parental support of grown children. *Journal of Marriage and Family, 74*(4), 880–896. https://doi.org/10.1111/j.1741-3737.2012.00987.x

Fingerman, K. L., Huo, M., & Birditt, K. S. (2020). A decade of research on intergenerational ties: Technological, economic, political, and demographic changes. *Journal of Marriage and Family*, *82*(1), 383–403.

Fingerman, K. L., Pitzer, L. M., Chan, W., Birditt, K., Franks, M. M., & Zarit, S. (2010). Who gets what and why? Help middle-aged adults provide to parents and grown children. *Journals of Gerontology Series B: Psychological Sciences and Social Sciences*, *66*(1), 87–98. https://doi.org/10.1093/geronb/gbq009

Gilbert, L. (2019). *Why people with intellectual disability experience lower life expectancy: Study*. Retrieved October 7, 2020, from https://medicalxpress.com/news/2019-12-people-intellectual-disability-life.html

Green, S. E. (2007). We're tired, not sad: Benefits and burdens of mothering a child with a disability. *Social Science and Medicine*, 64(1), 150–163. https://doi.org/10.1016/j.socscimed.2006.08.025

Healthwise Staff. (2020). *Family life cycle*. Retrieved June 9, 2021, from uofmhealth.org/health-library/ty6171#ty6172

Hunter, S. C., Riggs, D. W., & Augoustinos, M. (2017). Hegemonic masculinity versus a caring masculinity: Implications for understanding primary caregiving fathers. *Social and Personality Psychology Compass*, *11*(3), e12307. https://doi.org/10.1111/spc3.12307

Kim, Y.-I., & Swan, I. (2019). Religious heterogamy, marital quality, and paternal engagement. *Religions*, *10*(2), 102. https://doi.org/10.3390/rel10020102

Koenig, H. G. (2008, December 3). *How religious beliefs and practices are related to stress, health and medical services* [Paper]. Heritage Foundation Symposium.

Kripke, C. (2018). Adults with developmental disabilities: A comprehensive approach to medical care. *American Family Physician, 97*(10), 649–656.

Landes, S. D., & Settersten Jr., R. A. (2019). The inseparability of human agency and linked lives. *Advances in Life Course Research*, *42*. https://doi.org/10.1016/j.alcr.2019.100306

Lee, J. Y., & Lee, S. J. (2016). Caring is masculine: Stay-at-home fathers and masculine identity. *Psychology of Men and Masculinity, 19*(1), 47–58. https://doi.org/10.1037/men0000079

Lucas, J W., Greenberg, M., & Beavan, K. (2018). Research on physical disability in sociological social psychology: The state of the field and future directions. *Sociology Compass, 12*(2), e12555. https://doi.org/10.1111/soc4.12555

Lye, D. N. (1996). Adult child–parent relationships. *Annual Review of Sociology, 22*(1), 79–102. https://doi.org/10.1146/annurev.soc.22.1.79

Marsack, C. N., & Perry, T. E. (2018). Aging in place in every community: Social exclusion experiences of parents of adult children with autism spectrum disorder. *Research on Aging, 40*(6), 535–557. https://doi.org/10.1177/0164027517717044

McLaughlin, J. (2017). The medical reshaping of disabled bodies as a response to stigma and a route to normality. *Medical Humanities, 43*(4), 244–250. https://doi.org/10.1136/medhum-2016-011065

Molton, I. R., & Yorkston, K. M. (2017). Growing older with a physical disability: A special application of the successful aging paradigm. *The Journals of Gerontology: Series B, 72*(2), 290–299. https://doi.org/10.1093/geronb/gbw122

National Disability Navigator Resource Collaborative. (2020). *Population specific fact sheet—Intellectual disability.* Retrieved October 7, 2020, from https://nationaldisabilitynavigator.org/ndnrc-materials/fact-sheets/population-specific-fact-sheet-intellectual-disability/#:~:text=There%20are%20over%207%20million,or%20in%20the%20childhood%20years

National Down Syndrome Society. (2021). *Down Syndrome facts.* Retrieved June 29, 2021, from https://www.ndss.org/about-down-syndrome/down-syndrome-facts/

Nomaguchi, K., & Milkie, M. (2020). Parenthood and well-being: A decade in review. *Journal of Marriage and Family, 82*, 198–223. https://doi.org/10.1111/jomf.12646

Nowakowski, A. C. H. (2016). You poor thing: A retrospective autoethnography of visible chronic illness as a symbolic vanishing act. *The Qualitative Report, 21*(9), 1615–1635.

Oliver, M. (1996). Defining impairment and disability: Issues at stake. In C. Barnes & G. Mercer (Eds.), *Exploring the divide* (pp. 29–54). The Disability Press.

Ong, B. K. (2012). Grounded Theory Method (GTM) and the Abductive Research Strategy (ARS): A critical analysis of their differences. *International Journal of Social Research Methodology, 15*(5), 417–432. https://doi.org/10.1080/13645579.2011.607003

Parker, K., & Livingston, G. (2018). *Seven facts about American dads.* Pew Research Center. Retrieved May 19, 2019, from http://www.pewresearch.org/fact-tank/2018/06/13/fathers-day-facts/

Parsons, T. (1975). The sick role and the role of the physician reconsidered. *Health and Society, 53*(3), 257–278. https://doi.org/10.2307/3349493

Pleck, J. H. (2012). Integrating father involvement in parenting research. *Parenting,* 12(2–3), 243–253. https://doi.org/10.1080/15295192.2012.683365

Putnam, R. D. (2000). *Bowling alone.* Simon and Schuster.

Ricci, L. A., & Hodapp, R. M. (2003). Fathers of children with Down's Syndrome versus other types of intellectual disability: Perceptions, stress and involvement. *Journal of Intellectual Disability Research, 47*(4–5), 273–284. https://doi.org/10.1046/j.1365-2788.2003.00489.x

Roy, K. (2014a). Fathering from the long view: Framing personal and social change through life course theory. *Journal of Family Theory and Review, 6*(4), 319–335. https://doi.org/10.1111/jftr.12050

Roy, K. (2014b). Fathers on the frontiers of family change. *Journal of Family Theory and Review, 6*(1), 91–96. https://doi.org/10.1111/jftr.12031

Saldaña, J. (2011). *Fundamentals of qualitative research.* Oxford University Press.

Schoppe-Sullivan, S. J., & Fagan, J. (2020). The evolution of fathering research in the 21st century: Persistent challenges, new directions. *Journal of Marriage and Family, 82*(1), 175–197. https://doi.org/10.1111/jomf.12645

Seltzer, M. M., Floyd, F., Song, J., Greenberg, J., & Hong. J. (2011). Midlife and aging parents of adults with intellectual and developmental disabilities: Impacts of lifelong parenting. *American Journal on Intellectual and Developmental Disabilities, 116*(6), 479–499. https://doi.org/10.1352/1944-7558-116.6.479

Seltzer, J. A., & Bianchi, S. M. (2013). Demographic change and parent-child relationships in adulthood. *Annual Review of Sociology, 39*, 275–290. https://doi.org/10.1146/annurev-soc-071312-145602

Senior, J. (2014). *All joy and no fun: The paradox of modern parenthood.* Harper-Collins.

Smith, B., & Sparkes, A. C. (2016). Interviews: Qualitative interviewing in the sport and exercise sciences. In B. Smith & A. C. Sparkes (Eds.), *Routledge handbook of qualitative research in sport and exercise* (pp. 103–123). Routledge.

Special Olympics. (2021). *Our mission.* Retrieved June 19, 2021, from https://www.specialolympics.org/about/our-mission?locale=en

Stelle, C. D., & Sheehan, N. W. (2011). Exploring paternal maturity in the relationships between older fathers and adult children. *The International Journal of Aging and Human Development, 72*(1), 45–65. https://doi.org/10.2190/AG.72.1.c

Thoits, P. A. (2011). Mechanisms linking social ties and support to physical and mental health. *Journal of Health and Social Behavior, 52*(2), 145–161. https://doi.org/10.1177/0022146510395592

Thomas, P. A., Liu, H., & Umberson, D. (2017). Family relationships and well-being. *Innovation in Aging, 1*(3), 1–11. https://doi.org/10.1093/geroni/igx025

Timmermans, S., & Tavory, I. (2012). Theory construction in qualitative research: From grounded theory to abductive analysis. *Sociological Theory, 30*(3), 167–186. https://doi.org/10.1177/0735275112457914

Tomlinson, M., Yasamy, M. T., Emerson, E., Officer, A., Richler, D., & Saxena, S. (2014). Setting global research priorities for developmental disabilities, including intellectual disabilities and autism. *Journal of Intellectual Disability Research, 58*(12), 1121–1130. https://doi.org/10.1111/jir.12106

Turner, B. S. (2001). Disability and the sociology of the body. In G. L. Albrecht, K. D. Seelman, & M. Bury (Eds.), *Handbook of disability studies* (pp. 252–266). Sage Publications.

Turner, J. H. (1991). *The structure of sociological theory* (5th ed.). Wadsworth Publishing Company.

Umberson, D., & Karas Montez, J. (2010). Social relationships and health: A flashpoint for health policy. *Journal of Health and Social Behavior, 51*(S), S54–S66. https://doi.org/10.1177/0022146510383501

Umberson, D., Pudrovska, T., & Reczek, C. (2010). Parenthood, childlessness, and well-being: A life course perspective. *Journal of Marriage and Family, 72*(3), 612–629. https://doi.org/10.1111/j.1741-3737.2010.00721.x

The U.S. National Archives and Records Administration. (2021). *Previous sessions of Congress public law numbers.* Retrieved June 16, 2021, from https://www.archives.gov/files/federal-register/laws/past/106-second-session.txt

Verbrugge, L. M., & Jette, A. M. (1994). The disablement process. *Social Science and Medicine, 38*(1), 1–14.

Verbrugge, L. M., & Yang, L.-S. (2002). Aging with disability and disability with aging. *Journal of Disability Policy Studies, 12*(4), 253–267.

Videlefsky, A. S., Reznik, J. M., Nodvin, J. T., Heiman, H. J. (2019). Addressing health disparities in adults with developmental disabilities. *Ethnicity and Disease, 29*(Suppl 2), 355–358. https://doi.org/10.18865/ed.29.S2.355

Wilcox, W. B. (2004). *Soft patriarchs, new men: How Christianity shapes fathers and husbands.* University of Chicago Press.

Williams, S. (2008). What is fatherhood? Searching for the reflexive father. *Sociology, 42*(3), 487–502. https://doi.org/10.1177/0038038508088837

Zola, I. K. (1972). Medicine as an institution of social control. *The Sociological Review, 20*(4), 487–504. https://doi.org/10.1111/j.1467-954X.1972.tb00220.x

Zola, I. K. (1991). Bringing our bodies and ourselves back in: Reflections on a past, present, and future 'medical sociology.' *Journal of Health and Social Behavior,* 32, 1–16. https://doi.org/10.2307/2136796

CHAPTER 8

Life Course Eating Disorder Recovery on the Margins

Nik M. Lampe

As a medical sociologist, I have built an academic career in reading, writing, and discussing health disparities research—particularly concerning the needs and experiences of lesbian, gay, bisexual, transgender, queer, intersex, and asexual (LGBTQIA+) aging communities in the United States (U.S.). However, as a patient who has been in and out of eating disorder treatment and recovery centers for over a decade, this chapter was difficult to write for me. I never thought I would be alive long enough to write this autoethnography as an eating disorder survivor.

Eating disorders are multifaceted disturbances in eating and eating-related behaviors, thoughts, and practices that often affect one's health and quality of life (Williams, Russell-Mayhew, & Ireland, 2018). Estimates vary on how many people manage eating disorders due to existing stigma and ongoing academic and medical debates surrounding diagnosis criteria (i.e., what constitutes someone with eating disorder symptoms), but about 29 million Americans will manage an eating disorder in their lifetime (Deloitte Access Economics, 2020). Eating disorders can affect everyone regardless of age, race, ethnicity, nationality, class, sex, gender, and sexuality. Additionally, people of all sizes can live with an eating disorder. Eating disorder symptoms can occur during various stages of the life course, such as adolescence or older adulthood (Schaumberg et al., 2017). However, research and public discourse surrounding eating disorder diagnosis, management, and recovery have mostly focused on the experiences of young, white, non-Latin, thin, financially advantaged, heterosexual, endosex female, and cisgender women—leaving those who do not fit into these social dimensions with limited structurally-competent health resources, care, and support (zamantakis & Lackey, 2022).

I fall both within and on these margins as a patient-scientist who experiences intersecting forms of privilege and oppression (Crenshaw, 1989; Nowakowski, Sumerau, & Lampe 2020). I am a white, non-Latin, currently middle-class, transgender, non-binary, and intersex person in my late-20s who was assigned female at birth and raised as a cisgender woman in a rural, working-class neighborhood in the Midwestern U.S. I was diagnosed with anorexia at

 | DOI:10.1163/9789004708136_009

15 and then was diagnosed with bulimia at 16 and have been managing and recovering from eating disorder symptoms since 2009. I have sought treatment with five intensive inpatient and outpatient eating disorder recovery centers from 2009 to 2019. I have also attended hundreds of eating disorder support groups and individual therapy sessions during the past decade. I was hospitalized four times during adolescence due to eating disorder complications, such as experiencing severe dehydration, irregular heartbeats caused by electrolyte imbalances, stomach pain and bleeding, and iron deficiency anemia. Despite these health and healthcare needs, I struggled to find structurally competent eating disorder facilities and resources that were affirming of LGBTQIA+ and working-class patients. Thus, there is a critical need for revitalizing sociomedical research and practice in serving eating disorder patient populations on the margins. Using autoethnographic data, this chapter focuses on how principles of the life course perspective help illuminate eating disorder recovery on the margins and offer future directions in research.

1 Life Course Perspective

To further examine the eating disorder recovery experiences of underserved patient populations, it is important to understand how these communities manage their health and aging over the life course, so medical systems, facilities, and providers can create structurally competent practices in offering quality, effective care to eating disorder patients. Utilizing a life course perspective allows researchers to analyze macro and meso-level social pathways that define sequences of events, transition roles, and experiences of aging individuals and communities over time (Elder & Giele, 2009).

For example, sociomedical scientists have called for further expansion in the methods, theories, and empirically based evidence of investigating the lived experiences of transgender and non-binary people managing eating disorders and how instances of cissexism from medical providers and staff negatively impact their healthcare and quality of life (Nowakowski, Sumerau, & Lampe, 2020; zamantakis & Lackey, 2022). Health and aging both co-operate as social processes which occur over the life course and are often shaped by one's new understandings of the social world (Lampe, 2022; Nowakowski, Sumerau, & Lampe, 2020). Therefore, studying eating disorder patients from intersectionally marginalized communities while using a life course perspective offers fruitful avenues for researchers to further understand how these underserved communities in healthcare navigate social passages and life events over time concerning eating disorder diagnosis, management, treatment, and recovery.

Five major principles shape a life course perspective: (i) the interplay of time and place, (ii) life-span development, (iii) the timing of lives, (iv) human agency in choice making, and (v) linked lives (Elder, 1994; Elder, Johnson, & Crosnoe, 2003).

2 Time and Place

The interplay of *time and place* influences the social conditions of human lives (Elder, 1994), especially in the case of chronic illness management among socially and medically underserved communities (for examples see Lu et al., 2010; MacLean & Elder, 2007; Smith, 2007). From the perspectives of patients, family care partners, and medical providers, emerging research illuminates how the COVID-19 pandemic has substantially impacted eating disorder communities across the globe (Linardon et al., 2022; Weissman, Bauer, & Thomas, 2020). Many eating disorder patients, for example, have experienced and/or continue to experience substantial delayed or limited access to care services, resources, and support during the COVID-19 pandemic (Hamilton et al., 2022; Kaye & Bulik, 2021; Linardon et al., 2022). Therefore, when assessing eating disorder recovery resources during the COVID-19 pandemic, understanding the crucial interplay of time and place is a fundamental element in research on eating disorder patient populations.

During the COVID-19 pandemic, I experienced both barriers and facilitators to accessing care for my continued eating disorder recovery efforts. Recently after the World Health Organization declared the COVID-19 outbreak a global pandemic in 2020, medical providers on my recovery team were suddenly overwhelmed with an influx of patients needing immediate health services and support. My medical providers were only able to see and provide care for patients in crises. I also lived in central South Carolina at the time, which had an existing shortage of local specialty providers and facilities. Thus, I was suddenly unable to access the recovery care I needed from eating disorder specialty clinics and providers for over six months. Managing my chronic illness symptoms during a global emergency quickly became physically and emotionally taxing. At the time, I felt that I did not have the support I needed to continue meeting my eating disorder recovery goals. Due to COVID-19 national, state, and local lockdown measures, my family care partners were also unable to provide in-person care during that time. Such factors became setbacks in my eating disorder recovery efforts.

The COVID-19 pandemic also created facilitators that aided in improving my eating disorder management and symptoms. Living alone and social distancing during the first year of the pandemic created an environment where I was not frequently misgendered, navigating gender-segregated spaces (e.g., restrooms), or harassed in public settings for how I looked as a trans and non-binary person. Being trans and/or non-binary in a society that collectively believes and operates under a "cisgender reality" challenges the notion that sex and gender are fixed, limited, and stagnant social categories (Sumerau, Cragun, & Mathers 2016). Internalizing these repeated instances of cissexism can substantially impact the mental health and well-being of trans and non-binary people over the life course, which can be a major barrier to long-term eating disorder recovery efforts (zamantakis & Lackey, 2022). My eating disorder symptoms via cycles of extreme overeating (i.e., bingeing) and purging drastically reduced during COVID-19 because of the decline of cissexism in my personal and professional life. Future research should explore how the COVID-19 pandemic shapes the barriers and facilitators of care among eating disorder patients from intersectionally marginalized and privileged social locations.

3 Life Span Development

The *life span development* principle illustrates how people socially, psychologically, and physiologically develop in meaningful ways throughout adulthood via new trajectories, transitions, and conditions (Elder, 1994; Elder, Johnson, & Crosnoe, 2003). Approaches of and experiences with new situations throughout adulthood shape life span development individually (Elder & Giele, 2009) and collectively (Bockting et al., 2016). Prior lived experience vis-à-vis interactions with medical providers and staff, for example, have shaped my substantive training as a patient-scientist and advocacy work in bettering eating disorder treatment opportunities. The knowledge I have accumulated—along with my class privilege and resources—has helped me streamline my eating disorder treatment plan and tactics.

Through my Ph.D. coursework, I learned about the conceptualization of patient compliance (Ross, 1991) and my own realization that I do not have to comply with medically unnecessary norms during patient-provider interactions (e.g., weighing a patient who needs medical attention for a broken arm). Despite some pushback, I now opt out of disclosing my weight and allowing medical staff to weigh me during most appointments. Maintaining my mental health is more important to me than documenting my weight (when it is medically unnecessary) during clinical encounters.

Although scientific, medical, and public discourse prioritizes young eating disorder patients (Burke et al., 2020), emerging research suggests that life span development in mid-life and older adulthood considerably influences eating disorder management (Samuels, Maine, & Tantillo, 2019). Eating disorder symptoms and severity can also fluctuate or stay consistent across the life course (Fichter, Quadflieg, & Hedlund, 2006). The life span development principle is essential to understanding how eating disorder symptoms can exacerbate health and healthcare disparities at each life course transition, even in older adulthood. Future research should expand empirical knowledge, methods, and theories for accessing the needs and experiences of older adults at risk for or currently managing disordered eating.

4 Timing of Lives

The *timing of lives* principle highlights how the chronological timing of events and experiences may affect people's social expectations and beliefs over the life course (Bengtson, Elder, & Putney 2005; Elder, 1994). In the case of eating disorder survivorship, there may be ageist expectations for a patient to significantly reduce, eliminate, or better manage their eating disorder symptoms in older adulthood versus early adulthood (Peat, Peyerl, & Muehlenkamp, 2008). These assumptions in mainstream discourse contradict longitudinal data, which notes that admission to inpatient eating disorder facilities rates for American women 45 years or older have significantly increased in recent years and now account for 25% of admissions (Zhao & Encinosa, 2011).

If eating disorder management experience is chronologically out of sequence with age-related normative expectations in U.S. society (e.g., an older person with an eating disorder diagnosis or symptoms), such situations may act as a barrier or structurally disrupt older patients' access to structurally competent care resources, support, and services (Brandsma, 2007). When I have participated and engaged in eating disorder support groups in recent years, I have been told by both medical professionals and patients that I'm "too old" or "too experienced" to continue seeking eating disorder treatment and recovery services. Thus, social timing is influential in eating disorder recovery over the life course.

5 Human Agency in Choice Making

The *human agency in choice making* principle emphasizes the importance of how people's decision-making choices and processes influence their life course trajectories (Elder, 1994). Decisions shape our positionality in social situations, which may have immediate, short-term, and long-term consequences (Bengtson, Elder, & Putney, 2005; MacLean & Elder, 2007). At the same time, social resourcefulness (or lack thereof) also shapes human agency in decision-making processes and outcomes (e.g., no or limited health insurance coverage) (Smith, 2007), especially among medically and socially underserved communities in U.S. society (Lu et al., 2010). Human agency is an especially important element in the case of how eating disorder patient populations manage their health.

Medical authorities play a powerful role in enhancing or diminishing patients' feelings of control and human agency (Ross, 1991). I distinctly remember a horrific dining experience that I and other patients had at an outpatient eating disorder treatment facility while I was a master's student in Florida. The facility staff verbally abused and harassed us (e.g., calling us worthless, aggressively pulling on our hair and clothing, and threatening to transfer us to the inpatient care unit) and convinced us into eating all of the food on our plates within a 30-minute timeframe. We did not have the option of selecting our food or eating food with a fork, knife, or napkin. We also could not use the restroom by ourselves without being accompanied by staff (i.e., to avoid purging). If we did not eat all of the food on our plates, we would be forced to drink a large protein shake that had a disgusting taste and smell. The staff would also weigh us in front of everyone in the group before and after we ate. Such sociomedical contexts reproduce a lack of human agency in choice-making and feelings of control among patients, which may delay progress in achieving eating disorder treatment and recovery goals.

6 Linked Lives

The *linked lives* principle—a central element in life course research (Elder, 1994)—underscores how human lives are not fully independent, but socially "linked" or integrated with others from social relationships, networks, and influences (Halfon & Hochstein, 2002; Settersten, 2015). Social linkages go beyond formal relationships and often shape individual and collective interpretations of the social world (Mayer, 2009). For example, many eating disorder patients have family care partners (i.e., family caregivers) who help them better manage their chronic health conditions (Anastasiadou et al., 2014). Eating disorder patients and their family care partners both contribute to maintaining their social linkages, which may further influence life course pathways. Social linkages can also be maintained, discontinued, and disrupted over the life course, such as the COVID-19 pandemic disrupting prior community care partnerships and responsibilities. Little research explains how eating disorder patients' social relationships and support systems have changed during the COVID-19 pandemic and how such changes shape their health management possibilities and strategies.

7 Discussion

Using a life course perspective (Elder, 1994; Elder & Giele, 2009), I focused on how a life course perspective provides a valuable, conceptual foundation for illuminating the care needs, access, and utilization experiences among eating disorder patients from intersectionally marginalized and privileged social locations. I further pinpoint which specific barriers and resources I drew upon to adequately maintain my recovery efforts, which meaningfully informs medical providers and staff of opportunities for improvement in providing structurally competent care to eating disorder patients. Finally, I illustrate how principles of the life course perspective apply to eating disorder management, treatment, and recovery on the margins.

Such findings have the potential to enhance intervention research on eating disorder recovery and survivorship. Eating disorder patients from socially and medically underserved communities often experience greater challenges in managing their health due to intersectional marginalization in the forms of racism, classism, ageism, sexism, heterosexism, and cissexism (Burke, Schaefer, Hazzard, & Rodgers, 2020; Crenshaw, 1989). Consequently, eating disorder patient populations continue to experience health and healthcare inequities in later life (Fredriksen Goldsen et al., 2019). Thus, researchers and clinicians need to be culturally responsive while tailoring their research studies, skills-training, and support interventions to the needs of eating disorder patients from older, racial and ethnic minority, financially disadvantaged, and LGBTQIA+ communities.

References

Anastasiadou, D., Medina-Pradas, C., Sepulveda, A. R., & Treasure, J. (2014). A systematic review of family caregiving in eating disorders. *Eating Behaviors*, *15*(3), 464–477.

Bengtson, V. L., Elder, G. H., Jr., & Putney, N. M. (2005). The life course perspective on aging: Linked lives, timing and history. In M. L. Johnson (Ed.), *The Cambridge handbook of age and ageing* (pp. 493–501). Cambridge University Press.

Bockting, W., Coleman, E., Deutsch, M. B., Guillamon, A., Meyer, I., Meyer III, W., Reisner, S., Sevelius, J., & Ettner, R. (2016). Adult development and quality of life of transgender and gender nonconforming people. *Current Opinion in Endocrinology, Diabetes, and Obesity*, *23*(2), 188–197.

Brandsma, L. (2007). Eating disorders across the life span. *Journal of Women & Aging*, *19*(1–2), 155–172.

Burke, N. L., Schaefer, L. M., Hazzard, V. M., & Rodgers, R. F. (2020). Where identities converge: The importance of intersectionality in eating disorders research. *International Journal of Eating Disorders*, *53*(10), 1605–1609.

Crenshaw, K. (1989). Demarginalizing the intersection of race and sex: A Black feminist critique of antidiscrimination doctrine, feminist theory, and antiracist politics. *University of Chicago Legal Forum*, *1989*(1), 139–167,

Deloitte Access Economics. (2020). *The social and economic cost of eating disorders in the United States of America: A report for the Strategic Training Initiative for the Prevention of Eating Disorders and the Academy for Eating Disorders.* https://www.hsph.harvard.edu/striped/report-economic-costs-of-eating-disorders/

Elder Jr., G. H. (1994). Time, human agency, and social change: Perspectives on the life course. *Social Psychology Quarterly*, *57*(1), 4–15.

Elder Jr., G. H., & Giele, J. Z. (2009). *The craft of life course research*. The Guilford Press.

Elder, G. H., Johnson, M. K., & Crosnoe, R. (2003). The emergence and development of life course theory. In J. T. Mortimer & M. J. Shanahan (Eds.), *Handbook of the life course* (pp. 3–19). Springer.

Fichter, M. M., Quadflieg, N., & Hedlund, S. (2006). Twelve-year course and outcome predictors of anorexia nervosa. *International Journal of Eating Disorders*, *39*(2), 87–100.

Halfon, N., & Hochstein, M. (2002). Life course health development: An integrated framework for developing health, policy, and research. *The Milbank Quarterly*, *80*(3), 433–479.

Hamilton, A., Mitchison, D., Basten, C., Byrne, S., Goldstein, M., Hay, P., Heruc, G., Thornton, C., & Touyz, S. (2022). Understanding treatment delay: Perceived barriers preventing treatment-seeking for eating disorders. *Australian & New Zealand Journal of Psychiatry*, *56*(3), 248–259.

Kaye, W. H., & Bulik, C. M. (2021). Treatment of patients with anorexia nervosa in the US—A crisis in care. *JAMA Psychiatry*, *78*(6), 591–592.

Lampe, N. M. (2022). Liminal lives in uncertain times: Health management during the COVID-19 pandemic among transgender and non-binary older adults. *Gerontology and Geriatric Medicine*. https://doi.org/10.1177/23337214221127753

Linardon, J., Messer, M., Rodgers, R. F., & Fuller-Tyszkiewicz, M. (2022). A systematic scoping review of research on COVID-19 impacts on eating disorders: A critical appraisal of the evidence and recommendations for the field. *International Journal of Eating Disorders*, *55*(1), 3–38.

Lu, M. C., Kotelchuck, M., Hogan, V., Jones, L., Wright, K., & Halfon, N. (2010). Closing the Black-White gap in birth outcomes: A life-course approach. *Ethnicity & Disease*, *20*(1 Suppl 2), 62–76.

MacLean, A., & Elder Jr., G. H. (2007). Military service in the life course. *Annual Review of Sociology*, *33*(1), 175–196.

Mayer, K. U. (2009). New directions in life course research. *Annual Review of Sociology*, *35*(1), 413–433.

Nowakowski, A. C. H., Sumerau, J. E., & Lampe, N. M. (2020). *Transformations in queer, trans, and intersex health and aging*. Lexington Books.

Peat, C. M., Peyerl, N. L., & Muehlenkamp, J. J. (2008). Body image and eating disorders in older adults: A review. *The Journal of General Psychology*, *135*(4), 343–358.

Ross, F. M. (1991). Patient compliance—Whose responsibility? *Social Science & Medicine*, *32*(1), 89–94.

Samuels, K. L., Maine, M. M., & Tantillo, M. (2019). Disordered eating, eating disorders, and body image in midlife and older women. *Current Psychiatry Reports*, *21*(8), 1–9.

Schaumberg, K., Welch, E., Breithaupt, L., Hübel, C., Baker, J. H., Munn-Chernoff, M. A., Yilmaz, Z., Ehrlich, S., Mustelin, L., Ghaderi, A., Hardaway, A. J., Bulik-Sullivan, E. C., Hedman, A. M., Jangmo, A., Nilsson, I. A. K., Wiklund, C., Yao, S., Seidel, M., & Bulik, C. M. (2017). The science behind the academy for eating disorders' nine truths about eating disorders. *European Eating Disorders Review*, *25*(6), 432–450.

Settersten Jr., R. A. (2015). Relationships in time and the life course: The significance of linked lives. *Research in Human Development*, *12*(3–4), 217–223.

Smith, J. P. (2007). The impact of socioeconomic status on health over the life-course. *Journal of Human Resources*, *42*(4), 739–764.

Sumerau, J. E., Cragun, R. T., & Mathers, L. A. B. (2016). Contemporary religion and the cisgendering of reality. *Social Currents*, *3*(3), 293–311.

Weissman, R. S., Bauer, S., & Thomas, J. J. (2020). Access to evidence-based care for eating disorders during the COVID-19 crisis. *International Journal of Eating Disorders*, *53*(5), 639–646.

Williams, E. P., Russell-Mayhew, S., & Ireland, A. (2018). Disclosing an eating disorder: A situational analysis of online accounts. *The Qualitative Report*, *23*(4), 914–931.

zamantakis, a., & Lackey, D. (2022). Dying to be (a) gendered: An exploratory content analysis of trans/nonbinary people's experiences with eating disorders. *Sociological Inquiry*, *92*, 870–893.

Zhao, Y., & Encinosa, W. (2011). *An update on hospitalizations for eating disorders, 1999 to 2009: Statistical brief #120*. US Agency for Health Care Policy and Research.

CHAPTER 9

Still Living, Still Dying

Autoethnographic Inquiry on Aging with Cystic Fibrosis

Alexandra "Xan" C.H. Nowakowski

People who know my medical history generally ask me two questions: *How are you still alive?* and *Are you still dying?* The first question has always been rather difficult to answer. Lately, the second has as well. Ultimately, the answers to both are *I don't know*—with all the complications, qualifications, and inscrutabilities those words bring. Yet as little as I ultimately know about how I survived in the past or may continue to survive in the future, I have learned more than a few things along the way. This chapter is a reflection on that learning.

I am 36 years old, and I have a chronic disease called cystic fibrosis (CF). Once upon a time, these two things would not have belonged in a sentence together. When I was first being tested for CF, the median life expectancy for United States residents with this condition was about 10 years (Davis, 2006). By the time I got diagnosed conclusively, this number had increased to 37 years (Fajac & De Boeck, 2017). As I write this chapter, median life expectancy for people with CF is currently sitting at 47 years (CF Foundation). By the time I die, this number may look little different from my own age at that moment.

For those unfamiliar with CF, the disease can best be understood as follows. Every person has membranes in their body that secrete a liquid called mucus. This substance is usually thin and clear, allowing it to lubricate various organ tissues and help the body stay healthy overall. In people with CF, however, the mucus our bodies produce more closely resembles rubber cement in texture and consistency (Salvatore et al., 2017). As a result, it does not lubricate anything particularly well. Instead, our mucus often obstructs small passageways in our organs that help things get to where they need to be—like the enzymes our pancreases are supposed to release to help us digest our food. It also plays host to all kinds of bacteria and fungi that can do great harm to our internal organs.

Readers may at this point wonder why anyone's body would produce such a useless and ultimately harmful substance in the first place. Scientists are still figuring out exactly why this occurs, but have understood for several decades that a protein called the cystic fibrosis transmembrane conductance regulator (CFTR) impacts the texture and consistency of mucus (Vernon et al., 2017).

 | DOI:10.1163/9789004708136_010

People who do not have CF can make this protein, move it out of their cells, and use it appropriately once it gets to the surface. CF results from the body's inability to do one or more of these things. Whether or not a person can create, move, and use the CFTR protein depends largely on the coding of the genes that correspond to this protein. If something is out of sequence or just plain missing in one or both of these genes, a person will likely have at least some physical symptoms of CF.

Most people with CF have an improperly coded CFTR gene on both sides of their birth lineage (Cutting et al., 2019). However, some of us only have one mutation that interferes the functioning of our properly coded gene. In certain rare cases, problems with other genes can even affect how well the CFTR genes work. Yet whether we have two CFTR mutations, one, or none, those of us living with CF have something fundamental in common. As we get older, our health problems tend to become worse, and the vast majority of us will eventually die from something related to our underlying diagnosis. CF is thus classified as both a progressive disease and a fatal one. However, what actually kills us and when is a bit more complicated than all that.

As I write this chapter, statistics on causes of death among people with CF have not changed nearly as much as those on life expectancy. About 97% of people with CF will eventually die from the disease (Stephenson et al., 2017). Within that group, about 80% of people will die from respiratory failure. The other 20% will die from something else—kidney failure, liver failure, heart failure, etc. Failure is a common theme in the lives of people with CF, from our frequent early-life diagnoses of "failure to thrive" to the bizarrely hilarious scenario of experiencing "failure to die" if we survive beyond the allotted time for a hospice insurance benefit. So another common theme as we grow older is humor—often the darker the better.

I became interested in studying the nuances of aging with CF because I already had to deal with these things in my own life. In my typically sardonic and rather careerist way, I figured I might as well get some value out of having to struggle with perfunctory tasks like digesting food and getting oxygen. Eating and breathing are actually pretty easy for many adults with CF. In fact, we are often remarkably good at sucking down large quantities of food and huge lungfuls of air. What happens next is the problem: We get limited value out of pretty much anything that enters our bodies. Most of us take medications—pills, liquids, inhalers, nebulizers—to help our bodies overcome those challenges. Because CF affects a wide variety of systems, this adds up to a lot of medications and a lot of challenges…and consequently, a lot of stories.

Amplifying the stories of myself and other people aging with CF has tremendous value beyond the advancement of my own research program, of course. Although I began with the idea that autoethnographic inquiry might offer me an impactful means of making sense of my own experiences and thus some relief from the emotional pain I was feeling, it became something much bigger than that. I realized that by using my own story as a lens for gathering and interpreting data about the experiences of others from the CF community, I could fundamentally help to change people's understanding of how people with this disease age—and what we may need from others in the process. Aging with CF involves challenges in both clinical and social domains. I have found autoethnographic inquiry beneficial for understanding both sets of experiences, both individually and synergistically.

Explaining the clinical challenges of growing older with CF is relatively straightforward. Although the specific sets of challenges that individual patients experience as we age can vary somewhat, most of us will deal with some combination of lung and intestine issues, plus additional impacts to organs like our kidneys and livers, and at least some degree of both joint and immune problems (Bonk et al., 2017). My own aging process has involved terrible problems with my intestines and significant issues with my lungs; a variety of secondary impacts like exocrine failure, kidney disease, heart issues, sinus polyps, poor circulation, ruptured arteries, tooth loss, and gum damage; plus moderate arthritis and generalized autoimmunity.

These challenges tend to present for both early and late diagnosed people, as well as those who do not fit neatly into either category. I received a variety of incorrect and incomplete diagnoses along the way before finding out conclusively at age 32 that I really did have CF. The process to diagnose me began when I was much younger—around 5 years old—but failed to yield conclusive results because I could not produce a sufficient sample of sweat to get a valid screening test. I did not receive much in the way of coordinated CF care as a child, although my main doctor was fairly that I had the disease. Once I became an adolescent, I fell off the proverbial cliff and entered a long downward spiral that would not abate until I got diagnosed. Some of the more esoteric challenges I now face—such as losing several of my teeth and nearly all of my original gum tissue—owe in part to the copious damage done by my disease during the interim period between that initial suspicion and its confirmation. In other areas, my challenges are fairly typical.

Explaining the social challenges of aging with CF is perhaps less straightforward. Given the immense variety of contexts, values, histories, and goals that people bring to their interactions in the first place, it would be difficult to outline a remotely uniform social experience of growing older with CF. Indeed, the tremendous heterogeneity of personal biographies of aging in the CF community represents a unique opportunity for impact through autoethnographic inquiry. Yet in my initial forays into this topic, some common threads appeared with relative speed.

Some of these common themes from aging with CF as a specific social process began appearing in my general autoethnographic work on chronic illness nearly three years before I myself was formally diagnosed. By contrast, others emerged only when I became integrated into the CF community myself. At the time of my own conclusive diagnosis, I was already well aware of how general medical sociology concepts like the sick role, illness management, and biographical disruption were operating in my life and evolving as I aged (see Morden et al., 2017). I had comparatively less knowledge—and little personal context—for concepts specific to the experience of people with CF. Because there is very little sociological literature on any aspect of CF, and almost none on the process of aging with it, I can describe these themes only in the vernacular of the patient community itself.

I gathered information about and analyzed these social experiences—both the general ones and those specific to CF—in a process parallel to my own journey of discovery with my clinical status and care. I devote the remainder of this chapter to reflection on each of five successive autoethnographies of aging. As my own context shifted from a race against time with a mysterious disease that had almost killed me several times to a fully fledged war against a known disease that would almost certainly kill me one day, I journeyed deeper into the experiences and emotions of both myself and others with life-threatening chronic conditions. In the moment where I crossed the threshold from general illness to specific label, I realized I had a unique opportunity to conduct critical inquiry on aging with CF in both the pre-diagnosis and post-diagnosis stages.

My first autoethnography was called "Hope Is a Four-Letter Word: Riding the Emotional Rollercoaster of Illness Management" (Nowakowski, 2016a). It focused on the daily struggles and successes involved in managing chronic illness, rather than the moments of crisis in a health journey that much of the existing social science literature centered on at the time. I described the process of starting treatment for a specific subset of my symptoms that stemmed from intractable dry mouth, and of adjusting to that new treatment strategy. Several months before beginning the manuscript, I had been placed on the oral form of a drug called pilocarpine. I had begun using this drug in the hopes of mitigating my excessive thirst and the constant burning sensation in my mouth, as well as keeping my teeth healthier and preparing to undergo additional reconstructive surgeries on my gums. I was not yet using inhaled steroids for my lungs; that development would occur several months after my final gum surgery the following year.

Initially I got excellent results from the pilocarpine. I began to produce a substantial quantity of thinner saliva, and saw less of the white coating on my tongue that indicated large amounts of bacteria flourishing in my mouth. However, I soon began experiencing bizarre symptoms that perfectly matched with several of the side effects noted in the drug literature. These included bulging eyes, throbbing headaches, flank pain, stomach cramps, and excessive salivation. It took several rounds of adjusting my dosage with the pilocarpine itself, as well as identifying that I was consuming other substances through my diet that were irritating the tissue in my mouth and stomach, before my doctors and I settled on a functional strategy for giving me the benefits of the drug without so many side effects. I wound up on about one third of my original daily dosage. More than four years later, I continue to take the same low dose of pilocarpine each morning. I have found the drug to have numerous benefits beyond its stated aims. Because I take it orally, it helps with lubrication not only for the mucous membranes in my mouth but also for tissues elsewhere in my body.

The plot also thickens here somewhat: Pilocarpine is already familiar to many in the CF community, as the topical form of this drug is used in stimulating fluid secretion from the skin for chloride sweat testing. Some CF care providers are now experimenting with the oral form of the drug—as my team continues to—as an alternative to inhaled mucus thinning drugs like Pulmozyme whose benefits extend beyond the lungs. I was yet again becoming immersed in innovative therapeutics for CF despite not yet knowing for sure that I actually had the disease. I was also learning just how frustrating the daily changes people with CF experience with our health as we grow older can be. I built on the medical sociology literatures about "good days and bad days" and "hope and despair" that had begun to emerge in the early 2000s (Bister, 2018). In the process, I added perspectives about the unique complexities of living with a poorly understood illness and experiencing autoimmune symptoms. A particularly cruel reality of CF is how it can lead your body to attack itself as it grows older. I look back on that early work and continue to feel both impressed and haunted by what I learned in the process of analyzing my field notes for that first autoethnography.

Likewise, I quickly found myself thoroughly immersed in autoethnographic inquiry about the general experience of living with chronic illness. Many of the insights I was recording in my field notes for the "Hope Is a Four-Letter Word" manuscript ventured far outside of the conceptual boundaries of that particular exploration. Consequently, I began compartmentalizing my notes into thematic areas, separating those for the preliminary manuscript from ideas for additional inquiry. Several subtopics within my field notes coalesced around the dual concept of visibility and invisibility in chronic illness management. This content became the basis for my second autoethnographic study.

My second autoethnography was called "You Poor Thing: A Retrospective Autoethnography of Visible Chronic Illness as a Symbolic Vanishing Act" (Nowakowski, 2016b). It focused on the diverse ways in which I had experienced simultaneous feelings of visibility and invisibility as a person living and aging with chronic disease. In developing field notes for this paper, I ventured outside of my own internal experiences and thoughts to describe the behavior of others towards me in different settings. Using an interactionist framework, I explored how people defined the situation in interacting with me based on where they encountered me and what other factors shaped our meeting. My analyses of these experiences coalesced around a central theme of people both calling attention to and erasing the agency of people with visible chronic conditions by perceiving us as frail and ineffectual. I described how chronic illness became both a spotlight and a shadow in the lives of people living with it, and how these dynamics might evolve with continued aging (Spencer et al., 2017).

When I began compiling field notes for this project and writing the manuscript, I had still not yet received a conclusive diagnosis of CF, but had already learned ample information about the true scope and complexity of my disease. This made the study a distinct case of situated knowledge (see Haraway, 2004) because of its unique context in both personal biography and clinical information. My perceptions of the general embodied experience of living with visible chronic disease thus differed during those months from the insights I would share now in the context of CF specifically.

In addition to growing older chronologically in the period between submitting the "You Poor Thing" manuscript and seeing it published, I transitioned into the general contextual context of aging with CF. This overall process involved two key contextual transitions in specific domains of illness management. First, I transitioned from the context of an unknown disease to that of a known one. The inchoate feelings associated with experiencing significant health challenges in the absence of a coherent diagnosis gave way to both a profound sense of relief about my ability to get appropriate health care in the present, and highly specific fears about what the future might hold (Coyle & Atkinson, 2018). CF is both a manageable disease and a capricious one; the shift from one aspect to the other can mean death for someone who was recently thriving (Castellani & Assael, 2017). This is one of the core defining features of growing older with CF. Second, I transitioned from the context of a deviant body to that of a normative one. The same characteristics that made my body look unusual to others in absence of information about the underlying condition and how it might explain my physical appearance began to make it look much more usual once this information became known. Many adults with CF are very thin; this is so common that it has become a widespread stereotype of the condition.

Both of these contextual transitions thus helped both me and others to make sense of my experiences and how they presented visually. By the time I presented "You Poor Thing" at the 2017 annual conference for The Qualitative Report, I had already received a conclusive diagnosis of CF and begun the process of seeking coordinated care. I had not yet attended an office visit with an adult CF care provider, nor assembled a comprehensive care team. Yet the learning that occurred during this time period—both about my condition itself and how my view of my own aging process should evolve in response—lent a tremendous sense of coherence to what previously seemed a very dissonant and inscrutable biography of growing older with chronic disease (Helgeson & Zajdel, 2017). I would reflect on this evolution in my thinking, and how I was able to help my loved ones shift their own perspectives accordingly, in the process of publishing my third autoethnographic project.

My third autoethnography was called "Death Check: Doing Life and Research with Chronic Autoimmune Disease" (Nowakowski, 2017). It focused on documenting the complete timeline and progression of my symptoms as I aged from early childhood into young adulthood, and on contextualizing that journey within the broader scope of sociomedical science research on illness and identity across the life course. This inquiry populated a chapter for the volume about health research engaging personal biography that I was editing with my spouse at the time. We had proposed the book because we wanted to highlight a wide spectrum of experiences and contributions of scholars doing work informed by personal history of trauma. Chapters submitted by our collaborating authors covered a diverse array of topics, from racial injustice to biphobic violence to natural disaster, all with a shared focus on how these adverse experiences impacted the health of both research participants and scholars themselves.

When we began the process of proposing and compiling that edited volume, my spouse and I expected to look purely retrospectively at the lived experiences that informed our respective professional work. In my own chapter, focusing on the full life course perspective afforded a variety of valuable insights about aging with chronic illness and potential sources of social inequity associated with that overall experience (Frohlich & Potvin, 2009). Looking back over the 32 years I had lived at that point in time helped me to demonstrate that the relationship between illness and identity is neither static nor necessarily predictable after people receive and adjust to diagnoses (Oris et al., 2018). Rather, I illustrated in my own autoethnographic reflections that illness management is a dynamic process of constantly redefining and assimilating concepts of normalcy. Our approach to the book as a whole would soon took a different turn of its own, mirroring this general truth about illness management in aging individuals.

My spouse and I shifted our approach to framing the edited volume because I was definitively diagnosed with CF during the final stages of the manuscript preparation process. We thus developed a concluding chapter focused on both that unique moment in time and its implications for the future. The original chapter I had written remained unaltered; we saw value in illustrating the dynamic nature of illness management journeys as people age through structure as well as through content. In compiling my original chapter, I felt both cognizant of and ambiguous about the fact that my disease might actually be CF. This point had emerged in discussions with both my health care providers and my family members, but afforded no obvious course of action until I showed up at my primary doctor's office with a lurid purple rash covering much of my hips and thighs. A somber tone permeated that visit, as we both suspected the rash indicated significant damage to my kidneys and blood vessels. I did not know for sure yet that I had CF, but by then I knew at least some of my history with assessment for the disease, and the inconclusive nature of those results. My doctor sent me and my inch-thick chart file to a nearby hematologist who, without so much as making preliminary small talk, asked if I had ever been tested for CF.

That day, I began adjusting out of the possibility and into the probability that I had been living with CF my entire life, and thus growing older each day with the disease raging relatively unchecked in my body. This experience proved both frightening from an emotional perspective and fascinating from an intellectual one. I began incorporating this new information into my work with the reflection piece that concluded the edited volume on deeply personal health research. In the months that followed I continued to learn more about my condition, began receiving coordinated care, and integrated myself into the CF community. These experiences would later populate the field notes for my fourth autoethnographic study.

My fourth autoethnography was called "Neverland: A Critical Autoethnography of Aging with Cystic Fibrosis" (Nowakowski, 2019). It focused on the experiences of adjusting to the identity of CF patient, and planning for my future in the context of this illuminating yet unsurprising diagnosis. After I learned that I did indeed have CF, I reflected on spending the remainder of my lifetime both negotiating that identity and managing the underlying condition. As I was looking inward at my own hopes, fears, and goals I also began looking outward at the reactions of others to my diagnosis. I quickly realized that perceptions of CF in spaces both outside and within the patient community itself were often either incomplete or wholly inaccurate. The idea that people with CF do not grow old stood out as a common and especially problematic misconception, and thus formed the central conceptual framework for this new autoethnographic study.

Exploring this misconception and its likely origins led me to reflect on my own perpetual process of learning about where I fit within the general landscape of aging CF patients. When I first got my official diagnosis, I had thought I might be a relatively typical case of late diagnosis. I learned from both the scientific literature and other members of the CF community that late diagnosis of CF is relatively rare. I also learned that in cases where someone does get diagnosed well into adulthood, this usually occurs because the person only began experiencing symptoms as an adult, or encountered some hidden complication such as limited fertility (Sosnay et al., 2017). It would take over a year for me to meet anyone whose story mirrored my own. Learning how uncommon it was for people with mainstream physical presentations of the disease to survive for more than three decades without a conclusive diagnosis instilled two distinct sets of emotions within me about my continued journey of aging with CF. On the one hand, this information made me feel resilient about my past survival of adverse medical circumstances, and confident about my future ability to handle the additional challenges inherent in growing older with the disease. On the other hand, this information made me feel fearful about having lost too much time in my past care to rebound fully from the damage done by my CF during that time, and uncertain about what might happen in the future as a result of this delayed access to appropriate clinical services.

Conducting formal autoethnographic inquiry on the broad longitudinal process of aging with CF for the "Neverland" manuscript proved both illuminating and empowering, and enabled me to make a unique contribution to the sociomedical literature on chronic disease. However, it did not enable me to reflect in detail on the "daily grind" elements of illness management that inspired me to begin doing autoethnographic work in the first place. To achieve conceptual integration in my developing program of research on aging with CF, I needed to focus more closely on those small yet significant experiences of daily self-management. I thus began developing field notes for a fifth autoethnography using an entirely different type of source material.

My fifth autoethnography was called "Reframing Health and Illness: A Collaborative Autoethnography on the Experience of Health and Illness Transformations in the Life Course" (Nowakowski & Sumerau, 2019). It focused on my overall process of adjustment to managing my CF in the present and planning for my potential needs in the future through the lens of my daily experiences.

To achieve this level of detail, I used my own social media posts as the source material for the project. I also enlisted the help of my spouse, a highly experienced ethnographer, to help me achieve a more nuanced perspective on my own writings. This marked my first foray into both detailed autoethnography of self-management as someone growing older with CF, and collaborative ethnographic inquiry drawing simultaneously on the perspectives of patient and caregiver.

The collaborative approach to ethnography used in the "Reframing Health and Illness" study demanded a unique methodological strategy. I began by compiling a comprehensive archive of my own Facebook posts with the hashtag "#CFAdventures" over a one-year time period, arranging the material in chronological order. I then sent this archive, which contained approximately 60 single-spaced pages of text, to my spouse for review. They made their own field notes on the source material I had provided, then compared their insights with my own from reviewing the posts.

In preparing this fifth autoethnography I delved deeply into both my daily activities for managing my CF and my overarching sense of identity as a person aging with the disease. This approach enabled me to capture detailed information about the wide variety of elements involved in routine self-management for CF, and to contextualize that information within the broader evolution of identity that aging patients may experience. I learned quickly that aging with CF involves a perpetual dualism between learning and teaching roles—learning about your own condition through clinical assessment and perhaps also participation in academic research, and teaching others about the realities of living with the disease both in the present and over time. Indeed, my #CFAdventures posts on Facebook neatly encapsulated and showcased both of these processes—my own learning by writing them, and my teaching of others by sharing them.

I also learned that the teaching and learning processes implicated in growing older with CF necessarily involve constant reassessment of both a person's core identity and what is normal within the context of that identity. Aging with CF can perhaps be understood as a constant process of adjusting to a "new normal" in a situation where nothing at all is normal, and in which that sense of normalcy must remain extremely dynamic. Early on in my use of social media to share my #CFAdventures journey, I met another patient who was around my age and also deeply involved in public health research. We connected through a mutual friend without CF who had seen my posts and thought to make an introduction, and talked on the phone some two weeks afterwards. I found it wonderfully enriching to discuss my professional work and possible collaborations with another person who shared so many of my core perspectives. Yet by far the most affirming element of this exchange was the simple feeling of being completely normal in the presence of this other scholar. My sense of what my own future might look like changed dramatically after that day, in part because I opened my mind to the idea that I could seek support from and share ideas with other scientists aging with CF.

Engaging scientific research resources also helped me to make sense of my own personal biography more, and to envision my future with greater agency. In the summer of 2017, I agreed to have my full CFTR gene sequenced by a local laboratory. This process, which took several weeks, became the subject of multiple #CFAdventures posts. My results afforded insight into both why I might not have been able to produce consistent results on a chloride sweat screening, and why I was able to survive despite my extensive history of insufficient CF care. I found out that I had an extremely rare mutation (c.1584+36A<G) that had never before appeared in a US resident with CF. The prospect of being able to contribute new data to research proved exciting for both my own personal health care planning and my general advocacy for rare disease inquiry. I readily agreed to take two additional chloride sweat tests, both of which yielded a combination of insufficient samples and inconsistent results. Knowing both my genotype and my history of sweat screening performance enabled me to connect with CF researchers at Shands, who took an interest in studying my case history and aging process. This development enabled me to access my dual identity as scholar and patient in new ways, and frankly seemed like the ultimate adventure in growing older with CF (Lupton, 2017).

Transitioning from a framework of pure fear and anger into one of comingled empowerment and agency has certainly given me a more positive outlook on both my own prospects for continued aging with CF and those of the general patient community. Moreover, the processes of research inquiry that have facilitated this transition in my own life have given me a rich vocabulary for communicating these lessons to others within and beyond clinical settings (Ettore et al., 2017). For example, I now facilitate education for pediatric CF care providers about transitional care for younger patients who are aging into adulthood. I also work with nonprofit organizations to provide learning and sharing spaces for adult CF patients focused on healthy aging. In these ways and many more, my own critical inquiry on growing older with CF has enabled me to shape both cognitive and instrumental resources for other aging patients.

These inquiry projects have also done little to mitigate the essential duality in my own process of growing older with CF. I have aged more than three years since receiving a conclusive diagnosis, and experienced many improvements in both my health care resources and the benefits I obtain from engaging them. I have also continued to experience frightening phenomena with my physical health, and to manage the mental health implications of dealing with these experiences. I am thriving, which comes with both immense joy at the ground I have gained and immense fear at the prospect of losing it. At age 36 I am very much still living and still dying—still living despite a history of immense challenges, and still dying on an uncertain timetable. My autoethnographic explorations of aging with CF have demonstrated that both of these dynamics matter equally in the overall experience of growing older with this disease. Centering this consciousness in both further research inquiry on and evolving clinical care for CF represents a unique opportunity to improve quality of life in patients' individual and collective processes of aging.

References

Bister, M. D. (2018). The concept of chronicity in action: Everyday classification practices and the shaping of mental health care. *Sociology of Health & Illness, 40*(1), 38–52.

Bonk, M., Rey, M. M., & Hadjiliadis, D. (2017). New comorbidities in the changing face of cystic fibrosis care. *Journal of Cystic Fibrosis: Official Journal of the European Cystic Fibrosis Society, 16*(6), 647–648.

Castellani, C., & Assael, B. M. (2017). Cystic fibrosis: A clinical view. *Cellular and Molecular Life Sciences, 74*(1), 129–140.

Coyle, L.-A., & Atkinson, S. (2018). Imagined futures in living with multiple conditions: Positivity, relationality and hopelessness. *Social Science & Medicine, 198*, 53–60.

Cutting, G. R., Engelhardt, J., & Zeitlin, P. L. (2019). Genetics and pathophysiology of cystic fibrosis. In R. W. Wilmott, A. Bush, R. R. Deterding, F. Ratjen, & P. Sly (Eds.), *Kendig's disorders of the respiratory tract in children* (9th ed., pp. 757–768). Elsevier.

Davis, P. B. (2006). Cystic fibrosis since 1938. *American Journal of Respiratory and Critical Care Medicine, 173*(5), 475–482.

Ettorre, E., et al. (2017). *Health, culture and society: Conceptual legacies and contemporary applications.* Springer.

Fajac, I., & De Boeck, K. (2017). New horizons for cystic fibrosis treatment. *Pharmacology & Therapeutics, 170*, 205–211.

Frohlich, K. L., & Potvin, L. (2008). Transcending the known in public health practice: the inequality paradox: The population approach and vulnerable populations. *American Journal of Public Health, 98*(2), 216–221.

Haraway, D. (2004). Situated knowledges: The science question in feminism and the privilege of partial perspective. *Turning Points in Qualitative Research: Tying Knots in a Handkerchief, 2*, 21.

Helgeson, V. S., & Zajdel, M. (2017). Adjusting to chronic health conditions. *Annual Review of Psychology, 68*, 545–571.

Lupton, D. (Ed.). (2017). *Self-tracking, health and medicine: Sociological perspectives*. Routledge.

Marshall, B. C. (2017). *Survival trending upward but what does this really mean?* Cystic Fibrosis Foundation. https://www.cff.org/CF-Community-Blog/Posts/2017/Survival-Trending-Upward-but-What-Does-This-Really-Mean/

Morden, A., Jinks, C., & Ong, B. N. (2017). Temporally divergent significant meanings, biographical disruption and self-management for chronic joint pain. *Health, 21*(4), 357–374.

Nowakowski, A. C. H. (2016a). Hope is a four-letter word: riding the emotional rollercoaster of illness management. *Sociology of Health & Illness, 38*, 899–915. https://doi.org/10.1111/1467-9566.12403

Nowakowski, A. C. H. (2016b). You poor thing: A retrospective autoethnography of visible chronic illness as a symbolic vanishing act. *The Qualitative Report, 21*(9), 1615–1635. https://doi.org/10.46743/2160-3715/2016.2296

Nowakowski, A. C. H. (2017). Death check: Doing life and research with chronic autoimmune disease. In A. C. H. Nowakowski & J. E. Sumerau (Eds.), *Negotiating the emotional challenges of conducting deeply personal research in health*. Routledge.

Nowakowski, A. C. H. (2019). Neverland: A critical autoethnography of aging with cystic fibrosis. *The Qualitative Report, 24*(6), 1338–1360. https://doi.org/10.46743/2160-3715/2019.3549

Nowakowski, A. C. H., & Sumerau, J. E. (2019), Reframing health and illness: A collaborative autoethnography on the experience of health and illness transformations in the life course. *Sociology of Health & Illness, 41*, 723–739. https://doi.org/10.1111/1467-9566.12849

Oris, L., et al. (2018). Illness identity in adults with a chronic illness. *Journal of Clinical Psychology in Medical Settings*, 1–12.

Salvatore, D., Buzzetti, R., & Mastella, G. (2017). Update of literature from cystic fibrosis registries 2012–2015. Part 6: Epidemiology, nutrition and complications. *Pediatric Pulmonology, 52*(3), 390–398.

Sosnay, P. R., et al. (2017). Diagnosis of cystic fibrosis in nonscreened populations. *The Journal of Pediatrics, 181*, S52–S57.

Spencer, G., Lewis, S., & Reid, M. (2017). Living with a chronic health condition: Students' health narratives and negotiations of (ill) health at university. *Health Education Journal*, 0017896917738120.

Stephenson, A. L., et al. (2017). Survival comparison of patients with cystic fibrosis in Canada and the United States: A population-based cohort study. *Annals of Internal Medicine, 166*(8), 537–546.

Vernon, R. M., et al. (2017). Stabilization of a nucleotide-binding domain of the cystic fibrosis transmembrane conductance regulator yields insight into disease-causing mutations. *Journal of Biological Chemistry, 292*(34), 14147–14164.

www.ingramcontent.com/pod-product-compliance
Lightning Source LLC
Chambersburg PA
CBHW071447230926
51846CB00001B/367
* 9 7 8 9 0 0 4 7 0 8 1 1 2 *